Aids to Undergraduate Medicine

Other title in the Aids series

Burton Aids to Postgraduate Medicine 6E
Burton Aids to Undergraduate Medicine 6E
Dixon Aids to Pathology 4E
Habel Aids to Paediatrics 3E
Habel Aids to Paediatrics for Undergraduates 2E
Hayes and MacWalter Aids to Clinical Examination 2E
Mead Aids to General Practice 3E
Mowschenson Aids to Undergraduate Surgery 4E
Rogers and Spector Aids to Clinical Pharmacology and Therapeutics 3E
Rogers and Spector Aids to Pharmacology 3E
Scratcherd Aids to Physiology 3E
Sinclair and Webb Aids to Undergraduate Obstetrics and Gynaecology 2E

For Churchill Livingstone:

Publisher: Laurence Hunter
Project Editor: Barbara Simmons
Copy Editor: Ruth Swan
Project Controller: Nancy Arnott
Design Direction: Erik Bigland

Aids to Undergraduate Medicine

J. L. Burton MD BSc FRCP
Professor of Dermatology
Bristol Royal Infirmary, Bristol

B. J. L. Burton MA MRCP
Senior House Officer
The National Hospital for Neurology and Neurosurgery, London

SIXTH EDITION

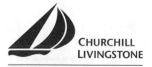

CHURCHILL
LIVINGSTONE

EDINBURGH LONDON MADRID MELBOURNE NEW YORK SAN FRANCISCO
AND TOKYO 1997

CHURCHILL LIVINGSTONE
Medical Division of Pearson Professional Limited

Distributed in the United States of America by Churchill
Livingstone Inc., 650 Avenue of the Americas, New York, N.Y.
10011, and by associated companies, branches and
representatives throughout the world.
© Longman Group Limited 1973
© Longman Group UK Limited 1990
© Pearson Professional 1997
The rights of J. L. Burton and B. J. L. Burton to be identified as
authors of this work have been asserted by them in accordance
with the Copyright, Designs and Patents Act 1988.

First edition 1973
Second edition 1976
Third edition 1980
Fourth edition 1984
Fifth edition 1990
Sixth edition 1997

ISBN 0 443 05692 7

British Library Cataloguing in Publication Data
A catalogue record for this book is available from the British
Library

Library of Congress Cataloging in Publication Data
A catalog record for this book is available from the Library of
Congress

Medical knowledge is constantly changing. As information
becomes available, changes in treatment, procedures,
equipment and the use of drugs become necessary. The author
and publisher have, as far as it is possible, taken care to ensure
that the information given in the text is accurate and up-to-date.
However, readers are strongly advised to confirm that the
information, especially with regard to drug usage, complies
with current legislation and standard of practice.

The
publisher's
policy is to use
paper manufactured
from sustainable forests

Produced by Longman Asia Ltd, Hong Kong
NPCC/01

Preface

This book is primarily intended to provide a compact aid to revision for candidates taking the final MB medicine examination, though candidates for other medical examinations may also find it helpful.

Many medical educators condemn learning by rote. Nevertheless, candidates in medical examinations still find it necessary to retain a formidable number of facts and we believe that the use of 'skeleton' lists as an adjunct to comprehensive textbooks can encourage an orderly approach to the subject as well as provide a basis for expansion in answers to examination questions.

It is impossible to achieve comprehensive coverage in a book of this size, but we have tried to select information which is worth remembering for use either in the assessment of common clinical situations or in reply to some of the more commonly asked examination questions. Many of the lists we have included are not readily available in the usual undergraduate textbooks, and for some important examination topics we have provided lists which are more detailed than those given in most undergraduate textbooks.

This sixth edition has been completely updated and a new feature is the introduction of mnemonics. The chapter on examination technique has also been expanded.

Bristol, 1997   J.L.B.
London, 1997   B.J.L.B.

Contents

1. Hints on the final MB medicine examination

Examinations are formidable even to the best prepared, for the greatest fool may ask more than the wisest man can answer.
Charles C Colton 1820. Lacon I: 322

The final MB examination is intended to prevent the qualification of incompetent doctors, and the examiners have the duty of ensuring that every successful candidate is safe to be 'licensed to heal'. They require to know that:

1. You have a sound knowledge of the basic principles of medicine and a common sense approach to the subject
2. You have had practical experience on the wards and can detect and interpret physical signs
3. You can prescribe safely, i.e. you know the mode of administration and approximate dosage of important drugs, and you know their main actions and serious side-effects
4. You can recognize and treat medical emergencies competently

Any candidate who satisfies the examiners on these points is fairly certain to pass the examination, but bear in mind the lugubrious corollary that if the examiners demonstrate a deficiency in these abilities, failure may follow.

REVISION

An important function of revision is to identify and eliminate 'blind spots'. Nobody can know everything, but you should aim to be completely ignorant about nothing, and the commoner the topic, the more you should know about it. A good way to cover topics which are likely to occur in the examination is to see as many cases on the wards as possible during your training and to 'read around' them. Most good physicians base their knowledge on cases they have seen personally, and it is quite a good idea as a student to keep a brief record of the patients you have seen as an aid to later revision.

A sound knowledge of medicine is obviously essential, but rapid recall of that knowledge in the exam is equally important. Instead of reading part of the textbooks in detail just before the exam, it's better to refresh your memory of the whole field, even if only in a superficial way. This will be facilitated if your lecture notes are all kept on loose-leaf paper of a standard size so that your knowledge from the various subspecialities can be integrated to avoid confusion and duplication of effort.

ESSAY QUESTIONS

The purpose of an essay question is to discover whether you can assemble your knowledge of a subject, select appropriate facts and opinions, arrange them in an orderly manner and then express yourself with clarity and good style. You should ask yourself what the examiners are trying to test in a particular question. They often have a fairly rigid marking code, awarding marks for each of certain predetermined points that are made, and no extra marks are awarded for even the most fascinating digressions. Candidates rarely fail final MB on the essay questions, but those who do are usually failed for not answering the questions that were asked.

Another cause for failure is misjudgement of the time allotted to each question. You should apply the 'law of diminishing returns' as it applies to essay questions — the first 40% for any question is easy, the next 30% is much harder, the next 20% is virtually impossible and the final 10% *is* impossible. Consistency in every question should be your aim. You should not, however, waste too much time on a question which you cannot answer. A blank simply scores no marks but an effusion of rubbish will prejudice the examiner against you.

Where possible, questions should be answered in terms of disturbance of physiology. This will demonstrate your knowledge of basic principles and also help you to arrange your answer in an orderly and rational manner.

Many candidates spend hours trying to predict questions by studying old papers. The syllabus is too big for this to be profitable in final MB, but it's worth checking the type of questions you'll be asked and spending time on any topics on which you are ignorant.

MULTIPLE-CHOICE QUESTIONS (MCQs)

You should familiarize yourself with the type of question favoured by your own medical school. Each question consists usually of five statements which are either true or false and you are required to give an answer of true, false or 'don't know' for each part. Typically a correct answer scores plus one, a wrong answer scores minus one and 'don't know' scores nothing. Exam papers often recommend answering only the questions you are sure of but if you did this you would probably end up only answering about 5% of the questions and failing. It is in the examiners' interest that people don't guess because the exam will then correctly select out the poor candidates; however, if all the poor candidates guess all the questions, some of them will pass who wouldn't otherwise have done so. It follows that there is an advantage to those candidates who answer more questions than others. If you find this hard to believe then try answering some practice papers, leaving questions out that you are unsure of and then repeating the paper answering all the questions as true or false. Most candidates will improve their score by between 1% and 10%. The important thing to remember is that you can fail by answering too few questions but you can't fail by answering too many, although you may still fail by being too ignorant. Remember too that the words 'always' and 'never' rarely apply to medicine and responses which contain them are unlikely to be true.

Another problem arises when a student has personally seen an unusual case which is the 'exception that proves the rule' and therefore has difficulty in answering an apparently simple question. This is a difficult dilemma, but in general it's probably best to ignore such personally-witnessed rarities unless you have seen them mentioned in standard textbooks.

Shortage of time is rarely a problem in MCQ exams and therefore answers can be checked. In our experience however 'second thoughts' in MCQ exams are rarely an improvement and we think it is preferable to work steadily through the paper once only, but noting any question which will require later thought.

THE CLINICAL EXAMINATION

Examiners rightly lay great stress on 'the clinical' when assessing a candidate and adequate preparation for this part of the examination is vital. The major skill required is of course the ability to elicit physical signs correctly but other factors such as fluency in case presentation and clinical judgement in the interpretation of the signs elicited are also important. The best way to improve your style in 'the clinical' is to obtain regular coaching from a critical senior colleague who will point out your faults. Failing this, you should make arrangements with a fellow student for each to see the other's cases under examination conditions. To obtain the maximum benefit you should of course 'grill' each other on the findings immediately afterwards. This method has the advantage that you will learn to see things from the examiner's point of view and you will quickly come to appreciate those bad habits which commonly cause annoyance to examiners.

Despite current trends, sartorial and tonsorial conservatism is recommended, as both patients and examiners are likely to be middle-aged if not actually senile.

THE MAJOR ('LONG') CASE

HISTORY-TAKING

A successful history demands just as much skill as the physical examination, and while two experienced clinicians will usually agree on the physical signs, the histories they obtain may be quite different. The examiners realize this and therefore attach more importance to the objective physical findings in assessing a candidate. An accurate history is important for diagnosis, however, particularly with cardiological or neurological patients, who are frequently used as 'long' cases because of their stable physical signs. There is more to the assessment of a cardiological case than merely hearing and interpreting the murmurs, which, contrary to popular belief, are usually 'loud and clear' in examination cases. It is vitally important to obtain the fullest possible details of previous illnesses, especially with regard to the duration, symptoms and treatment of any possible bouts of rheumatic fever, chorea, tonsillitis, SBE, etc., and in female patients you must obtain full details of previous pregnancies. Male patients can often give the results of previous medical grading prior to service in the armed forces, and many patients can give the date and result of previous chest X-rays. Details of the patient's past and present exercise tolerance are of course essential, and you should ascertain from the patient exactly how much physical effort his present work entails. In neurology cases the mode of onset (over minutes, days or weeks), length of history and subsequent course (static, steadily progressive or remitting) will usually suggest the type of pathological lesion present (e.g. vascular, inflammatory, neoplastic or degenerative), and the physical signs will then confirm the anatomical site of the lesion.

When taking a history in exams it is advisable first to list all the patient's symptoms briefly, to discover the type of illness and the systems involved. The symptoms should then be arranged chronologically and full details about each should be obtained. Thus if the patient complains of pain you should determine:
1. The site, with the direction of radiation
2. Its nature and severity
3. Its duration and periodicity
4. Any aggravating or relieving factors
5. Any associated features
Think about the possible diagnosis from the outset and modify your questions accordingly.

Never accept terms such as rheumatism and vertigo at their face value, but ask the patient what he means by this. You may be surprised, as was the GP who gave several prescriptions for bigger and better laxatives for an old dear who was 'costive', until he discovered she thought this was a synonym for diarrhoea.

Considerable persistence may be needed to prevent the patient digressing. With garrulous patients the previous medical and family histories are particularly difficult to obtain. In such cases stick to essentials and don't hesitate to ask leading questions in order to obtain the necessary information.

The history will allow you to assess the patient's mood, intellect, speech and memory, and you should of course observe the patient closely during the history for signs of dyspnoea, tremor, etc. It is also a good idea on first meeting the patient to ask yourself 'Could this be myxoedema?', as this diagnosis is otherwise easily missed.

Essential points of history-taking for the long case
- Name
- Age
- Occupation
- When was the patient last completely well?
- *Presenting complaint* and very thorough history of presenting complaint.
  — Ask about diseases related to the presenting complaint. For example if the suspected diagnosis is ulcerative colitis ask about possible complications such as erythema nodosum, pyoderma gangrenosum, eye involvement, joint problems, liver involvement, etc.
- *Past medical history*, particularly operations or previous hospital admissions.
  — Ask 'Have you ever had — high **B**lood pressure, heart attack (**MI**), **J**aundice, **T**uberculosis, **R**heumatic fever, **A**sthma, **D**iabetes, **E**pilepsy, **S**troke, **C**lots (DVT), peptic ulcer (**D**uodenal ulcer)? (Mnemonic = 'BMJ TRADES CD')
  — Also ask about sickle cell anaemia in all black patients and thalassaemia in all Mediterranean patients.
- *Drug history*
  — Ask why patients are on the medication they take.
  — Always ask about allergies, particularly to penicillin.
- *Family history*
  — Remember to ask about siblings as well as parents, grandparents and children. (Autosomal recessive conditions are unlikely to have occurred in previous generations but 'One of my three sisters has cystic fibrosis' provides a useful clue if your patient's presenting complaint is recurrent chest infections since childhood).
- *Social history*
  — Ask if the patient has ever smoked and if so for how long and why did they give up? 'I gave up when they found my lung cancer doc. Oops, I wasn't supposed to tell you that!'
  — Ask about alcohol consumption. Get details of how much and how often rather than accepting a glib answer such as 'only socially'.
  — Who is at home and are they able to look after the patient?
  — Does the patient have a district nurse, social worker, meals on wheels, telephone, stairs between him and the toilet? Who gets the shopping, does the housework, and can the patient wash himself?
  — Full occupational history, particularly for respiratory cases ('I spent two years removing asbestos from ships but that was 40 years ago').

— Do you have pets (particularly sick parrots)? What are your hobbies (e.g. pigeon fancier)?

System review
This is important as it should bring out any important information that the patient may have forgotten to tell you ('Oh, sorry, I thought you knew about the blood I'm coughing up. After all that's the real reason I'm here although as I was telling you my biggest problem is this terrible itch I get on my head every time I pass water').
Always ask about:
• Appetite.
• Weight loss — how much, over how long?
• *Respiratory system*. Shortness of breath (and when), wheeze, cough (productive?), haemoptysis (how much?), exercise tolerance (in metres or number of stairs).
• *Cardiovascular system*. Chest pain, palpitations (can you tap out the rhythm?), postural hypotension, orthopnoea, how many pillows do you sleep with, do you wake short of breath (PND or asthma), swelling of ankles.
• *Abdominal system*. Any dysphagia, reflux, indigestion, vomiting, haematemesis, abdominal pain? Bowel habit and any recent change? Diarrhoea (if so, how often and describe it), constipation, melaena, blood mixed in with stool or only on paper.
• *Genitourinary*
  — Nocturia or frequency (consider DM or UTI), incontinence, haematuria, offensive smell, poor stream, hesitancy, post micturition dribbling.
  — Previous pregnancies, heavy periods (consider anaemia and thyroid disorders), intermenstrual bleeding, recurrent abortions (antiphospholipid syndrome), premature menopause (consider other organ-specific autoimmune diseases).
• *Nervous system*. Fits, faints, visual disturbance, severe headaches, paraesthesiae, sensory loss, weakness, coordination.
• *General*. Skin problems, arthritis.

EXAMINATION

The ability to elicit and interpret physical signs is of course essential and considerable practice on the wards is required to achieve this skill. A combination of speed and thoroughness is required for exam purposes, and this applies especially to pulmonary percussion, cardiac auscultation and examination of the CNS. In auscultation in particular, first impressions are often right and prolonged listening may cause confusion. It's usually more convenient to examine a patient from the head downwards, rather than by systems, and regular practice with an unvarying routine is required if no major points are to be missed. We cannot stress too strongly that people fail their long case not through missing a minor abnormality, but because in their haste they have failed to look for a sign which is in fact present in a gross form. Obvious signs such as a large breast mass, hypertension, marked tracheal shift, gross optic atrophy, unilateral deafness, severe intention tremor, massive splenomegaly, etc., can easily be missed unless the appropriate examination is performed. Such signs may not always be suspected to be present from the history, although it is of course advisable to pay special attention to the systems where you expect positive findings. Thus it would be foolish to accept the absence of a mitral murmur too readily in a patient with dyspnoea, haemoptysis, and a malar flush, or to be satisfied with perfunctory palpation for splenomegaly in a patient with suspected leukaemia.

Equivocal findings can usually be safely ignored unless they are relevant to the symptoms or probable diagnosis. For example it is best not to waste much time over minor degrees of reflex inequality, slight facial asymmetry, impaired vibration sense, etc., unless your patient has a neurological disorder or a disease which causes a neuropathy. Other common causes of real or imagined equivocation which can often be ignored include slight bilateral pallor or blurring of the optic disc, slight tracheal or apical displacement, soft murmurs and slight inequality of breath sounds. Remember that small differences in percussion are easily imagined and bronchial breathing is uncommon. If a finding is dubious and it doesn't fit, forget it.

For the major case practise working well within the set time limit, so that you have time left at the end to recheck your positive findings and to look again for any associated signs which you might expect to be present in that particular case. Remember that mistakes in the history may occasionally be explained away as being due to the patient's poor memory, but mistakes in the physical signs are entirely the responsibility of the candidate and cannot be condoned.

On completion of the examination you should carefully consider the possible diagnoses and then clarify any doubtful points in the history. You should also amplify the history regarding any unexpected physical signs you have discovered.

Quite apart from any humanitarian considerations it is most important to try to establish a good rapport with your patient. Many of the patients used in the examination are chronic cases with more or less stable physical signs. Since such patients are in frequent demand for teaching purposes they usually have a long experience of young doctors and their difficulties and they are often well aware which of their own physical signs are commonly missed. Occasionally such patients will spontaneously volunteer valuable information with regard to their diagnosis or physical signs, but in other cases a judiciously worded question at the end of your examination such as 'Is there anything else you think I ought to know?' will often prove rewarding. Other useful clues may be obtained by asking the patient to describe the investigations and treatment he has had, and by asking him what he believes to be the cause of his symptoms. Occasionally you'll hit the jackpot with a reply such as 'Well the doctors at Queen Square said it was Frederick Attacks Yer'. You must be prepared for misleading answers however, and these should be ignored if they do not tally with your own assessment of the history and physical signs. These questions should be left until the end as otherwise the replies will prejudice your judgement. Another point to consider is that these questions sometimes provoke in the patient an uncooperative attitude of 'That's for me to know and you to find out' which can make subsequent history-taking difficult.

Before the examiner arrives you should reconsider your diagnosis and ask yourself 'Could this be anything else?' Remember that elderly patients often have multiple pathology, and remember too that although rare diseases occur rarely, their prevalence in examinations is greatly increased. If the diagnosis is uncertain prepare a list of different diagnoses and consider what investigations you would perform, remembering to mention simple tests such as ESR and chest radiograph before more expensive and possibly dangerous procedures. In most final MB exams, simple urine tests are required as part of the physical examination of the patient and this important step should not be forgotten. If there is time, you should consider how you would answer probable questions regarding management and prognosis, and in appropriate cases you should try to anticipate what the ECG and radiographs might show.

CASE PRESENTATION

There is quite an art in presenting a case concisely and clearly. The examiners have no time to waste, and hesitant and long-winded presentations are tedious, so you should edit the history, emphasizing important points, leaving out irrelevant detail and giving negatives only if they are important. If the case is straightforward the presentation of the history and examination should form a cohesive account leading to a confident diagnosis. In such cases try to make your assessment as full as you can and say whether the condition in your patient is acute or chronic, mild or severe, simple or with complications. In more difficult cases with conflicting evidence or doubtful signs you will have more reservations, but don't hedge all the time as this irritates examiners and does nothing to conceal your ignorance. Try to make up your mind on the basis of probabilities. Doctors often have to act on the basis of equivocal evidence and the examiners want to see whether you can take a sensible decision.

While it is important to keep your initial presentation concise, it is a mistake to answer the subsequent questions too curtly. The examiner is anxious to see whether you can discuss your patient intelligently and you should try to display your relevant knowledge as much as possible. If anything about the case puzzles you, or there is a problem relating to diagnosis or management, don't be afraid to acknowledge this. If the line of questioning seems to be entering one of your fields of ignorance, try to keep the initiative by talking around the subject. With a bit of luck you may introduce a fresh topic that interests the examiner. If he persists in reiterating a particular question this is often because he is trying to establish a very basic point. Examiners can be obtuse in the way they phrase such questions and prolonged silences in such circumstances can be disastrous. Try to talk sensibly around the subject to see what he's aiming at, and with luck a supplementary question will lead you to the required answer.

THE MINOR ('SHORT') CASES

Many students regard the minor cases as a little light relief from the more arduous parts of the examination. This is a serious misconception, for the examiners are well aware of the element of luck which enters into the major case, and they attach correspondingly greater importance to the candidate's performance while he is under direct observation. You will be watched as you examine the patient and your style in eliciting physical signs is important. Make a point of positioning the patient properly, and although you should preserve the patient's modesty as far as possible, remember that you may be penalized if you do not get the patient adequately undressed.

As in the long cases, a reasonable compromise must be reached between speed and thoroughness in physical examination, for as a general rule a candidate's score is proportional to the number of cases he has time to examine and diagnose correctly. It is obviously better to err on the side of over-caution rather than to fail because of a major error of omission, but remember that few things irritate an examiner more than the candidate who wastes time performing a tediously meticulous examination in what should be a simple, rapidly diagnosed condition. The examination of the sensory nervous system often provides cause for offence in this respect, and cardiological auscultation presents a similar hazard. If you are unsure of the diagnosis in a case with an 'interesting' murmur, there is usually no point in remaining glued to the patient's praecordium in the hope of being saved by the bell, for the examiner will certainly ask you for a diagnosis before dismissing you. Far better to think quickly, present a sensible differential diagnosis and move on to the next case.

Another important point in the minor cases is to listen carefully to the instructions of the examiner with regard to the part or system to be examined and obey them implicitly. Before recounting your findings however, you should always pause and ask yourself whether further examination of more distant parts of the body, such as regional lymph nodes, peripheral pulses, finger nails, etc., is required. If you are not clear what the examiner wants you to do, do not be afraid to ask for clarification. For example, if the examiner says 'Examine this patient's heart' it would be reasonable to ask whether he wishes you also to feel the pulse.

The importance of the recognition of clinical associations in the minor cases cannot be overemphasized. In many cases inspection of the patient and his immediate environment as you approach the bed may provide a clue to the diagnosis. For example you may be shown a cutaneous eruption localized to the shin in a patient with exophthalmos (pretibial myxoedema), or you may be asked to give the likely diagnosis of an arthritis in a patient who also has a patch of psoriasis, or marked nail pitting. The key to many minor cases lies in such observations and you should practise looking for such clinical associations until this becomes habitual.

Having elicited the physical signs correctly many candidates fail to be selective enough in applying their knowledge to the particular patient under discussion. Blind application of 'lists of causes' oblivious of the patient's age or sex, the associated physical findings, etc., are guaranteed to create a poor impression. The habit of mentioning rare diseases before common ones is another failing which is easily eradicated with practice.

Hints and tips received from earlier candidates in the short cases are on the whole best ignored. Examiners have been known to change the order of the patients' beds and they will certainly have changed the questions. There is moreover a real danger that you will jump to the diagnosis (which may in any case be wrong) without giving adequate consideration to the differential diagnoses and without eliciting the appropriate physical signs.

It is heartening to realize that for success in the clinical examination omniscience helps, but is by no means essential (indeed a few examiners seem to find it somewhat irritating). More important are adequate practice in examination technique, quick-wittedness, thoroughness, clear enunciation, a confident but modest bearing, and good luck.

THE ORAL EXAMINATION ('VIVA')

The 'viva' tests the depth as well as the breadth of a candidate's knowledge. If he appears to know a topic fairly well, the examiners will switch to another subject and if several common topics are satisfactorily dealt with, they may go on to test the candidate 'in depth'. For this reason, it may be worthwhile for the good candidate to learn about a few unusual multisystem conditions in detail and to try and introduce them into the conversation. For example a student who has spent an elective period in the USA might choose coccidioidomycosis as a subject to revise in detail. Then if he is asked about pneumonia, meningitis, osteomyelitis, tuberculosis, erythema nodosum or lymphadenopathy he will, after discussing the commoner causes, casually mention coccidioidomycosis. The examiner will often rise to the bait and say 'Ah yes, now what do you know about that?' The converse of this ploy is that you should not mention anything in the viva unless you're prepared to talk about it.

It is vital to have a good knowledge of the diagnosis and management of emergencies such as cardiac arrest, GI bleeds, MI, pulmonary oedema, drug overdoses, anaphylaxis and acute asthma. Don't worry too much about small print as no one will fail you for misdiagnosing pituitary apoplexy although they might if you fail to shock someone in ventricular fibrillation. (Recommended reading: *Acute medicine*, 2nd edition, by Springings, Chambers and Jeffrey, Blackwell Science.)

Students are often asked for the causes of a condition. Stony silence is not impressive. Even if you have never heard of the condition you can try the following sieve: TIN MAIDENS, which stands for **T**rauma, **I**nfection, **N**eoplasia, **M**etabolic (or Mechanical), **A**lcohol, **I**atrogenic (or Idiopathic), **D**egenerative (or Drugs), **E**ndocrine, **N**eurological, **S**moking. Infection can be broken down into viral, bacterial, fungal, protozoal and parasitic. Neoplasia should be considered as benign and malignant, primary and secondary. It sounds obvious but if you don't say it the examiner won't know that you know it.

It is worth remembering that some conditions such as AIDS, syphilis, TB, sarcoidosis, collagen–vascular disease and drug side-effects can occasionally cause almost anything.

You may be given a pathology specimen ('pot') to describe in the viva. Examine it carefully from all sides to try identify the organ first (not always easy), then describe the pathological lesions you can see, and hazard a diagnosis. If you know the answer try to talk at some length. If you haven't a clue, don't prevaricate but have a guess and go on to the next 'pot'. Tipping it upside down to look at the label is not recommended as it will only make the 'pot' too cloudy to see anything!

If you are shown a radiograph the abnormality is likely to be fairly gross, so stand back and take an overall view before looking at the details. Remember that more than one abnormality may be present (e.g. an absent breast shadow with pulmonary metastases, or a bronchial cancer with rib metastases), so examine the whole film. Assuming you can spot the abnormality it is best to discuss this from the outset as examiners get tired of being told that the patient is slightly rotated and the film is of poor quality.

Finally, have sympathy with your examiner. He cannot be expected to know everything and if you cross swords with him, give ground gracefully — after all he may be right!

2. Cardiology

CYANOSIS

5 g reduced Hb per 100 ml blood produces cyanosis. (Note that polycythaemic patients can be cyanosed without being hypoxic, and anaemic patients can be hypoxic without being cyanosed)

PERIPHERAL CYANOSIS

Due to poor peripheral circulation

Causes
1. Vasoconstriction, e.g. due to low ambient temperature or Raynaud's disease
2. Arterial obstruction, e.g. atheroma
3. Low cardiac output, e.g. failure, aortic stenosis

CENTRAL CYANOSIS

Due to low arterial oxygen saturation

Causes
1. Hypoventilation
2. Parenchymal lung disease
3. R to L cardiac shunt
4. Decreased PO_2 of inspired gas

   May be simulated by methaemoglobinaemia and sulphaemoglobinaemia

JUGULAR VENOUS PULSE (JVP)

Height of JVP is measured with reference to sternal angle with subject at 45° to horizontal
   Normally less than 4 cm (vertical height)

CAUSES OF ELEVATED JVP

1. R ventricular failure, esp. cor pulmonale, pulmonary embolus
2. Fluid overload (esp. i.v. infusion)
3. Tricuspid stenosis or incompetence
4. Pericardial effusion or constrictive pericarditis

5. Very slow heart rate, esp. complete heart block
6. Obstruction of superior vena cava (non-pulsatile)

Kussmaul's sign
JVP rises on inspiration. Seen in constrictive pericarditis, pericardial effusion, restrictive cardiomyopathy.

Normal jugular venous pulse wave in relation to ECG pattern

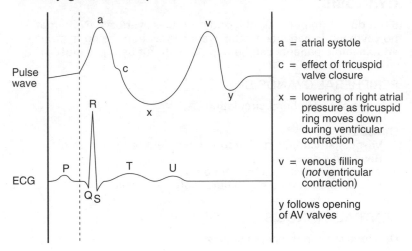

a = atrial systole

c = effect of tricuspid valve closure

x = lowering of right atrial pressure as tricuspid ring moves down during ventricular contraction

v = venous filling (*not* ventricular contraction)

y follows opening of AV valves

TYPES OF ARTERIAL PULSE WAVE

1. NORMAL

2. COLLAPSING (ALSO CALLED WATER-HAMMER OR CORRIGAN PULSE)

(i) Aortic incompetence
(ii) Hyperdynamic circulation (see p. 15)
(iii) Patent ductus arteriosus
(iv) Peripheral AV malformations

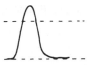

3. SMALL VOLUME

(i) 'Shock'
(ii) Aortic stenosis
(iii) Pericardial effusion

4. BISFERIENS

Combined aortic stenosis and incompetence

5. ANACROTIC (SLOW-RISING)

Aortic stenosis

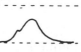

6. DICROTIC

Fevers

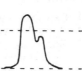

7. PULSUS ALTERNANS — Alternate strong and weak beats

Left ventricular failure

8. PULSUS PARADOXUS — Blood pressure decreases on inspiration by more than 10 mmHg

   (i) Pericardial effusion
  (ii) Constrictive pericarditis
 (iii) Severe asthma

ARTERIAL PULSE RATE

CAUSES OF TACHYCARDIA

1. Sinus tachycardia (q.v.)
2. Supraventricular (atrial or nodal) tachycardia
3. Atrial flutter (usually around 150/min)
4. Atrial fibrillation
5. Ventricular tachycardia (inc. torsade de pointes)
6. Ventricular flutter

CAUSES OF SINUS TACHYCARDIA (over 100 beats per minute)

1. Hyperdynamic circulation (q.v.)
2. Congestive cardiac failure
3. Hypovolaemic shock (acute haemorrhage, etc.)
4. Constrictive pericarditis
5. Drugs, e.g. adrenaline, atropine, salbutamol
6. Pulmonary embolism, asthma

CAUSES OF HYPERDYNAMIC CIRCULATION

1. Exercise or emotion (anxiety, fright, etc.)
2. Pregnancy

3. Anaemia
4. Pyrexia
5. Thyrotoxicosis
6. AV fistulae

CAUSES OF SINUS BRADYCARDIA (less than 60 beats per minute)

1. Extreme physical fitness
2. Convalescence from fever
3. Soon after myocardial infarction
4. Hypothyroidism
5. Hypothermia
6. Raised intracranial pressure (with hypertension)
7. Drugs, e.g. digitalis, beta-blockers
8. Sinoatrial disorder ('sick sinus syndrome')

CAUSES OF AN IRREGULAR PULSE

1. Extrasystoles
2. Atrial fibrillation
3. Marked sinus arrhythmia

COMMON CAUSES OF SOME ARRHYTHMIAS

EXTRASYSTOLES

1. Idiopathic
2. Fatigue, excessive smoking, alcohol or caffeine ingestion
3. Myocardial ischaemia
4. Digitalis
5. Hyperthyroidism
6. Heart diseases with atrial enlargement (e.g. mitral stenosis)

PAROXYSMAL TACHYCARDIA

1. Myocardial ischaemia
2. Digitalis, especially after potassium depletion

ATRIAL FIBRILLATION

1. Rheumatic heart disease, especially mitral stenosis
2. Myocardial ischaemia
3. Hyperthyroidism
4. Idiopathic 'lone fibrillation'
5. Mitral prolapse
6. Sick sinus syndrome
7. Hypertension

HEART BLOCK (all degrees)

1. Myocardial ischaemia
2. Digitalis
3. Chronic heart disease, especially aortic stenosis and congenital lesions
4. Rheumatic fever

CLINICAL DIAGNOSIS OF AN ARRHYTHMIA

1. SINUS ARRHYTHMIA

Rate *in*creases with *in*spiration

2. EXTRASYSTOLES (ectopic beats)

Atrial, nodal or ventricular
   (i) A premature beat with a compensatory pause followed by a stronger beat
   (ii) Usually runs of normal beats occur, but extrasystoles may alternate with normal beats (pulsus bigeminus)
   (iii) May disappear during exercise

3. ATRIAL FIBRILLATION

   (i) Completely irregular in time and force
   (ii) Worse on exercise
   (iii) Carotid compression has no effect
   (iv) JVP 'a' waves absent

4. ATRIAL FLUTTER

   (i) Regular radial pulse rate, classically 150/min in 2:l block (but can be irregular if there is fluctuating heart block)
   (ii) AV block occurs, so that the JVP 'a' waves greatly exceed the pulse rate
   (iii) Carotid compression slows the rate while pressure is maintained

5. PAROXYSMAL TACHYCARDIA

Atrial, nodal or ventricular
   (i) May be history of previous attacks with sudden onset and cessation
   (ii) Carotid compression may decrease the rate even after pressure is relaxed

6. HEART BLOCK

Complete (3rd degree)
Heart rate of 36–44/min which does not increase with exercise

2nd degree AV block
May be dropped beats (Wenckebach) or 2:1, 3:1 or 4:1 block.
Instability of rhythm is common

1st degree block
Detected only on ECG (PR > 0.2 second)

APEX BEAT — THE LOWEST AND OUTERMOST POINT OF DEFINITE CARDIAC PULSATION

Heart is enlarged or displaced if apex beat is:
1. Lateral to midclavicular line, or
2. Below 5th intercostal space
The character of the apex beat may be:
a. **Heaving** (pressure overload) in aortic stenosis or systemic hypertension (apex usually not displaced)
b. **Thrusting** (volume overload) in aortic regurgitation or mitral regurgitation (apex usually displaced)
c. **Tapping** ('palpable first heart sound') in mitral stenosis
   A left parasternal heave indicates RV hypertrophy

FAILURE TO LOCATE THE APEX BEAT ON PALPATION

Consider the following possibilities:
1. Excessively fat or muscular chest wall
2. Left pneumothorax, pleural effusion or emphysema
3. Large pericardial effusion
4. Dextrocardia or marked mediastinal shift
5. Massive LV hypertrophy. (Remember to feel as far round as the mid-axillary line)

THRILLS (palpable murmurs)

Always indicate an organic defect. The area localizes the defect

HEART SOUNDS

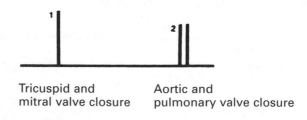

Tricuspid and   Aortic and
mitral valve closure   pulmonary valve closure

N.B.
1. Aortic normally closes before pulmonary

2. Pulmonary closure is delayed by inspiration (due to increased venous return caused by decreased intrathoracic pressure) The normal split therefore *in*creases on *in*spiration

FIRST SOUND

Loud in
1. Mitral stenosis
2. Hyperdynamic circulation
3. Tachycardia

Soft in
1. Mitral incompetence
2. Rheumatic carditis
3. Severe heart failure

SECOND SOUND IN AORTIC AREA

Loud in systemic hypertension
Soft in aortic stenosis

SECOND SOUND IN PULMONARY AREA

Loud in pulmonary hypertension (e.g. chronic pulmonary disease)
Soft in pulmonary stenosis

THIRD HEART SOUND

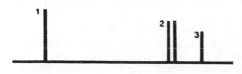

Heard at apex early in diastole, due to ventricular distension
Easily confused with opening snap of mitral stenosis which is maximal medial to the apex

Causes
1. Normal in young people and during pregnancy
2. Ventricular failure (a useful sign)
3. Mitral or tricuspid incompetence
4. Constrictive pericarditis

FOURTH HEART SOUND

Heard at lower end of sternum late in diastole, due to atrial contraction (and therefore not present in atrial fibrillation)

Always abnormal, indicates resistance to LV filling because of increased ventricular wall stiffness

Causes
1. Hypertension
2. Heart block
3. Myocardial infarction

   Triple rhythm is due to a 3rd or 4th heart sound, or summation of both

   Gallop rhythm is a fast triple rhythm, and indicates actual or incipient heart failure

   Dogmatic pronouncements on the state of the second sound and the presence or absence of the third and fourth sounds are not normally expected of undergraduates

CARDIAC MURMURS

When auscultating, concentrate separately on the heart rhythm, sounds and murmurs. The murmurs most commonly missed in exams are those of aortic incompetence and mitral stenosis. Aortic incompetence is missed either because auscultation was not performed all down the L sternal edge with the patient sitting up at the end of expiration, or because the candidate failed to 'tune in' to the high-pitched murmur. Mitral stenosis is missed either because the patient was not auscultated lying on his left side, or because the candidate listened to only one site in the apical area.

The examination of peripheral signs will give you an idea of what you might find on auscultation. For example if the patient is in atrial fibrillation consider mitral valve disease; then if the apex is displaced there is likely to be mitral regurgitation, otherwise a loud first heart sound and an undisplaced apex beat favour mitral stenosis.

If the patient is in sinus rhythm then the pulse character is useful, a slow rising pulse indicating aortic stenosis, a collapsing pulse indicating aortic regurgitation. Similarly if the apex is displaced then aortic regurgitation is much more likely than aortic stenosis. If the murmur radiates to the carotids aortic stenosis is more likely than mitral regurgitation, but the converse does not follow as the murmur of aortic sclerosis will not radiate to the carotids.

If there is a midline sternotomy scar there may be a prosthetic valve or two, in which case a systolic murmur may be normal. However most midline sternotomies are done for bypass grafting, not for valve replacement. None of these rules is absolute but they are useful.

If several murmurs are present, try to decide which lesion is dominant by consideration of associated clinical features, e.g. in simultaneous AS and AI the pulse may be either 'plateau' or 'collapsing', and in simultaneous MS and MI the presence of a 3rd heart sound with a soft 1st sound suggests the incompetence is dominant.

If no murmur is heard and the patient gives a history of rheumatic fever, you should exercise the patient and listen again, particularly for murmurs of MS or AI.

Differential diagnosis of murmurs

Timing	Maximal intensity	Likely causes
Ejection systolic	Aortic area	Aortic stenosis Aortic sclerosis Coarctation
	Pulmonary area	Innocent Pulmonary stenosis Atrial septal defect Pulmonary hypertension
	Apex	Innocent Aortic stenosis Aortic sclerosis
Pansystolic	Apex	Mitral incompetence Ventricular septal defect Fallot's tetralogy
		Tricuspid incompetence
	Lower sternal border	Ventricular septal defect
Mid-diastolic	Apex	Mitral stenosis
	Lower sternal border	Tricuspid stenosis (rare)
Diastolic	Anywhere along sternal border	Aortic incompetence Pulmonary incompetence
Continuous	Cardiac base	Patent ductus arteriosus Simultaneous AS and AI
	Above clavicle	Venous 'hum'

Remember the possibility of extracardiac sounds such as a pericardial rub in pericarditis

In any patient in whom you suspect rheumatic heart disease you should obtain details of the symptoms, duration and treatment of any previous bouts of possible rheumatic fever, chorea, tonsillitis or bacterial endocarditis.

CHARACTERISTICS OF INNOCENT SYSTOLIC MURMURS IN CHILDHOOD

1. No other abnormality detected (no cardiac enlargement)
2. No thrill or added sound
3. Never diastolic or pansystolic, except for the continuous murmur of a venous hum, which is reduced on lying down
4. Intensity often varies with a change in posture

MITRAL STENOSIS

Nearly always due to rheumatic heart disease, but rarely may be congenital

SYMPTOMS

1. Progressive exertional dyspnoea
2. Other symptoms of pulmonary congestion:
   (i)   Orthopnoea
   (ii) Paroxysmal nocturnal dyspnoea
   (iii) Cough
   (iv) Haemoptysis
3. Acute pulmonary oedema, usually precipitated by exertion, pregnancy or onset of AF
4. Recurrent bronchitis
5. In later stages, symptoms of RV failure (p. 27)
6. Palpitations in paroxysmal AF

SIGNS

1. Thin face with purple cheeks ('mitral facies')
2. Pulse may be small volume. May be atrial fibrillation
3. BP shows low pulse pressure
4. May be 'tapping' apex beat and L parasternal heave
   May be diastolic thrill
5. 1st heart sound is loud and 'slapping'
   2nd heart sound is loud if pulmonary hypertension is present
   May be 'opening snap' (indicates mobile valve) in early diastole
6. Rough, rumbling, low-pitched diastolic murmur, localized to the apical area and accentuated by exercise. May be presystolic crescendo if fibrillation absent
7. Pulmonary crackles
8. In later stages, signs of RV failure

N.B. Increased severity of stenosis is indicated by increased duration of murmur (not its loudness).

COMPLICATIONS

1. Thrombi in L atrium, and systemic embolization
2. Pulmonary emboli
3. Subacute bacterial endocarditis (uncommon with atrial fibrillation)

ELECTROCARDIOGRAM

1. May be broad notched P wave (L atrial hypertrophy)
2. May be atrial fibrillation
3. R axis deviation or R ventricular hypertrophy
4. Usually digitalis effects

MITRAL INCOMPETENCE

CAUSES

1. Mitral valve prolapse (usually myxoid degeneration)
2. Rheumatic fever (probably around 20% of cases in UK)
3. Ischaemia, especially posterior infarct, with papillary muscle damage
4. Subacute bacterial endocarditis (may be cause or complication)
5. Functional MI due to stretched AV ring in LVF

SYMPTOMS

1. Palpitations and exertional dyspnoea occur early
2. Fatigue and weakness
3. Orthopnoea due to pulmonary oedema

SIGNS

1. L ventricular dilatation
2. 1st heart sound is soft and muffled
   3rd heart sound is usual
3. Loud pansystolic murmur, maximal at apex and propagated to axilla
   Often obscures 2nd heart sound
4. May be LV failure

N.B. Increased severity is indicated by 3rd heart sound, LVF and a displaced apex

AORTIC STENOSIS

CAUSES

1. Congenital, particularly bicuspid valve (presents at age 40–60)
2. Rheumatic fever
3. Senile calcification of an otherwise normal valve (presents over 60)
4. Severe hypercholesterolaemia

SYMPTOMS

1. May be none for years
2. Symptoms of L ventricular failure (p. 26)
3. Syncope on effort
4. Angina (despite normal coronary arteries)

SIGNS

1. Small volume, slow-rising pulse
2. L ventricular hypertrophy
   May be systolic thrill (best felt with patient sitting forward at end of expiration)
3. 2nd sound in aortic area is soft
4. Harsh systolic 'ejection' murmur maximal at aortic area and radiating to the neck
5. May be LV failure

N.B. Increased severity is indicated by a slow-rising pulse, an inaudible second heart sound and a low BP.

Aortic sclerosis murmur is identical, but is distinguished by normal pulse wave and absence of a thrill!

AORTIC INCOMPETENCE

CAUSES

A. Valvar
1. Rheumatic fever
2. Subacute bacterial endocarditis
3. Bicuspid valve
4. Rheumatoid disease

B. Aortic root disease
1. Type A aortic dissection
2. Syphilis
3. Marfan's
4. Seronegative arthritis (p. 143)

SYMPTOMS

1. May be none for many years

2. Palpitations and dizziness
3. Symptoms of L ventricular failure (p. 27)
4. Angina

SIGNS

1. Collapsing (Corrigan) pulse. May be visible carotid pulsation or 'head-nodding' (de Musset's sign) or nail bed pulsation (Quincke's sign)
2. BP shows wide pulse pressure
3. L ventricular hypertrophy and dilatation
4. Murmurs:
   (i) Soft high-pitched blowing diastolic murmur down L sternal edge
   (ii) May be a systolic aortic murmur due to increased blood flow
   (iii) May be a diastolic apical murmur (Austin Flint) which simulates mitral stenosis
   (iv) May be 'pistol-shot' noise over femorals synchronous with pulse (Traube's sign)
   (v) May be diastolic murmur over femorals on slight compression with stethoscope bell (Duroziez's sign)
5. May be LV failure

N.B. Increased severity is indicated by *decreased* duration of murmur, LVF and a displaced apex

TRICUSPID INCOMPETENCE

CAUSES

1. Infective endocarditis (esp. in drug addicts)
2. Pulmonary hypertension
3. Rheumatic fever
4. Functional TI due to stretched AV ring in RVF
   Clinical manifestations usually determined by coexisting and predominating mitral stenosis

SYMPTOMS

1. Exertional dyspnoea is common, but orthopnoea and paroxysmal nocturnal dyspnoea are uncommon due to diminished R ventricular output into lungs
2. Gastrointestinal upsets due to venous congestion of GI tract

SIGNS

1. Elevated JVP with large v waves
2. Pulsatile hepatic enlargement
3. Ascites, which is both chronic and recurrent

4. Peripheral oedema, pleural effusions
5. Pansystolic murmur, maximal near lower sternum, and becoming louder during deep inspiration

CLASSIFICATION OF CONGENITAL HEART DISEASES
CYANOTIC (I.E. R TO L SHUNT)

1. Fallot's tetralogy
     (i) Pulmonary stenosis
    (ii) Ventricular septal defect
   (iii) Over-riding aorta
    (iv) Right ventricular hypertrophy
2. Transposition of great vessels and tricuspid atresia are usually fatal in infancy unless corrected
3. Eisenmenger's syndrome (reversal of a L to R shunt following the development of pulmonary hypertension)

ACYANOTIC

1. With L to R shunt
     (i) Ventricular septal defect
    (ii) Atrial septal defect — usually secundum but rarely septum primum
   (iii) Persistent ductus arteriosus
   These patients may become cyanosed due to cardiac failure, pulmonary infection, severe exercise or shunt reversal

2. With no shunt
     (i) Coarctation of aorta
    (ii) Pulmonary stenosis — occasionally cyanosed
   (iii) Congenital aortic stenosis
    (iv) Dextrocardia
     (v) Bicuspid aortic valves

HEART FAILURE

Definition: a state in which the heart fails to meet the metabolic and oxygen needs of the body under varying conditions, assuming the venous return is adequate

LEFT VENTRICULAR FAILURE

Common causes
1. Myocardial ischaemia
2. Hypertension
3. Aortic stenosis or incompetence
4. Mitral incompetence

Symptoms
1. Exertional dyspnoea
2. Orthopnoea
3. Paroxysmal nocturnal dyspnoea, often with coughing or wheezing
4. Pulmonary oedema (anxiety, dyspnoea, cough and pink frothy sputum)

Signs
1. Tachycardia. May be pulsus alternans
2. Enlarged heart
3. Gallop rhythm
4. May be functional mitral incompetence due to stretched AV ring
5. Fine crackles at lung bases. May be wheezes

LEFT VENTRICULAR HYPERTROPHY

Causes
1. Hypertension
2. Mitral incompetence
3. Aortic stenosis and/or incompetence
4. High output states, e.g. anaemia, polycythaemia, thyrotoxicosis
5. Aortic coarctation
6. Hypertrophic cardiomyopathy

Signs
1. Forceful apex beat, left ventricular heave
2. Loud aortic 2nd sound
3. Signs of any underlying condition

RIGHT VENTRICULAR FAILURE

Common causes
1. Secondary to L ventricular failure
2. Mitral stenosis
3. Cor pulmonale (including pulmonary embolism)
4. Congenital heart disease

Symptoms
1. Tiredness, weakness, anorexia
2. Oedema
3. Gastrointestinal upset. May be hepatic pain

Signs
1. Dependent oedema
2. Elevated JVP
3. May be functional tricuspid incompetence due to stretched AV ring

4. Large tender liver. May be mild jaundice
5. Oliguria by day and nocturia. Urine is concentrated and albuminuria is common
6. Peripheral cyanosis or ascites in severe cases
   Remember that R and L sided heart failure often appear almost simultaneously

SYSTEMIC HYPERTENSION

Definitions vary but 140/90 mmHg for a young adult and 160/95 mmHg for a middle-aged person would be reasonable upper limits

CAUSES

1. Essential
2. Renal disease (especially renal ischaemia)
3. Drugs, e.g. cyclosporin, oral contraceptives, glucocorticoids
4. Alcoholism and/or sleep apnoea
5. Endocrine
   (i)   Cushing's disease
   (ii) Phaeochromocytoma
   (iii) Primary aldosteronism (Conn's)
6. Coarctation (but BP normal in legs)
7. Toxaemia of pregnancy

COR PULMONALE

Cardiac disease secondary to chronic disease of lungs or pulmonary vessels

CAUSES

1. Emphysema and chronic bronchitis
2. Pulmonary fibrosis
3. Multiple pulmonary emboli
4. Severe kyphoscoliosis
5. Idiopathic pulmonary hypertension

SIGNS OF COR PULMONALE

1. Warm cyanosed extremities with bounding pulse
2. Raised JVP, hepatomegaly and oedema
3. Triple rhythm and loud P2 due to pulmonary hypertension (but overlying emphysema may cause soft heart sounds)
4. Functional tricuspid incompetence in severe cases

CAUSES OF SEVERE CHEST PAIN

1. Myocardial ischaemia
    (i) Coronary atheroma, thrombus or vasospasm
    (ii) Aortic valve disease or aortitis
    (iii) Severe anaemia
    (iv) Paroxysmal tachycardia
2. Pericarditis
3. Pleurisy
4. Pulmonary embolism
5. Oesophageal pain (acid reflux, spasm, carcinoma)
6. Expanding aortic aneurysm
7. Chest wall lesions
    (i) Rib fracture
    (ii) Metastatic deposits in ribs or fractures
    (iii) Myalgia (e.g. Bornholm disease)
    (iv) Herpes zoster
    (v) Idiopathic costochondritis (Tietze's syndrome)
8. Gastric or duodenal ulcer
9. Gallbladder colic or pancreatitis
10. Pain referred from thoracic or cervical spine

COMMON RISK FACTORS FOR MYOCARDIAL INFARCTION

1. Smoking
2. Hypertension
3. Hypercholesterolaemia
4. Diabetes mellitus
5. Family history of atheroma
6. Increasing age
7. Male sex

COMPLICATIONS OF MYOCARDIAL INFARCTION

EARLY (IN FIRST 48 H)

1. Cardiac arrhythmia
    (i) Sinus or nodal bradycardia
    (ii) Supraventricular tachycardia, atrial flutter, atrial fibrillation
    (iii) Ventricular ectopic beats, tachycardia, flutter or fibrillation
    (iv) Heart block
    (v) Cardiac asystole
2. Ventricular failure
3. Hypotension or 'shock'
4. Pericarditis
5. Ruptured papillary muscle or chordae tendineae
6. Ventricular septal defect
7. Iatrogenic (pacing, etc.)

MEDIUM (AFTER 48 H)

1. DVT, pulmonary embolism
2. Mural thrombosis, systemic embolism
3. Cardiac rupture (often after several weeks)

LATE (AFTER SEVERAL WEEKS)

1. Cardiac aneurysm
2. Dressler's syndrome due to cardiac autoantibodies (fever, chest pain, pericarditis or pleurisy)
3. Psychological, including 'L chest pain'
4. Frozen shoulder and 'shoulder hand' syndrome

CLINICAL 'SHOCK'

Definition: a syndrome in which inadequate blood supply and elimination of tissue metabolites lead to functional and/or structural disturbances in the essential organs

CAUSES

1. Hypovolaemia — haemorrhage, trauma, dehydration, burns, post surgery
2. Cardiac failure
   (i)   Pump failure, e.g. myocardial infarct
   (ii) Arrhythmia
   (iii) Obstruction, e.g. pulmonary embolism
3. Sepsis
4. Anaphylaxis

PERICARDITIS

CAUSES

1. Myocardial infarct
2. Viral (Coxsackie, Echo, etc.)
3. Rheumatic fever
4. Pyogenic (pneumonia or septicaemia)
5. Tuberculous
6. Cancer invading the pericardium (bronchus or breast)
7. Severe uraemia
8. SLE, rheumatoid disease
9. Dressler's syndrome

CONTRA-INDICATIONS TO THROMBOLYTIC THERAPY

1. Recent haemorrhage, trauma or surgery
2. Bleeding diathesis
3. Aortic dissection
4. Severe hypertension
5. Recent cerebro-vascular event (CVA)
6. Peptic ulcer
7. Heavy vaginal bleeding
8. Acute pancreatitis
9. Severe liver disease, esp. oesophageal varices
10. Pulmonary disease with cavitation
    Streptokinase or anistreplase should not be given again within 12 months of a previous dose, or if there was an allergic reaction

RHEUMATIC FEVER

Diagnosed by the revised *Jones' criteria*,
i.e. evidence of previous streptococcal infection plus either 2 major criteria or 1 major and 2 minor criteria from the following list:

MAJOR

Sydenham's chorea
Polyarthritis (migratory)
Erythema marginatum
Carditis
Subcutaneous nodules (painless)
Mnemonic — SPECS

MINOR

Pyrexia
ECG shows prolonged PR interval
Arthralgia
C reactive protein (or ESR) raised
History of previous rheumatic fever
Mnemonic — PEACH

3. Electrocardiography

THE NORMAL ELECTROCARDIOGRAM

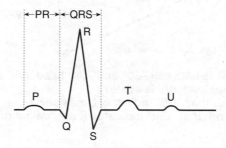

PR should be < 0.20 seconds
QRS should be < 0.12 seconds
1 large square (5 mm) on ECG, paper = 0.2 seconds

$\therefore$ Ventricular rate/minute = $\dfrac{300}{\text{No. of large squares between adjacent R peaks}}$

STANDARD LEADS

ECG interpretation is facilitated by imagining that the standard leads 'look at' the electrical activity of the heart from the following viewpoints in a coronal plane:

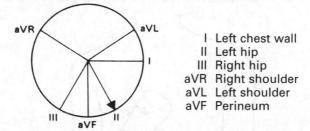

I Left chest wall
II Left hip
III Right hip
aVR Right shoulder
aVL Left shoulder
aVF Perineum

The cardiac axis can be worked out from leads I and aVF, remembering that R waves represent the direction of the vector

(Left ventricular depolarization) and S waves represent the opposite direction.

Summate R and S for each of these 2 leads.

Then height of R minus depth of S for lead I represents the vector in the horizontal direction, and height of R minus depth of S for lead aVF represents the vector in the vertical direction. A simple scale drawing of these two vectors then gives the cardiac axis:

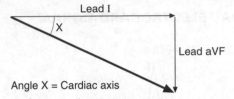

Angle X = Cardiac axis

The normal axis is between −30° and +90° (lead aVL is at −30°, lead I is at 0, and lead aVF is at +90°)

An axis of less than −30° indicates L axis deviation

An axis of more than +90° indicates R axis deviation

CHEST LEADS

These leads 'look at' the heart in a horizontal plane from the right of the sternum (**V1**) to the axillary line (**V6**)

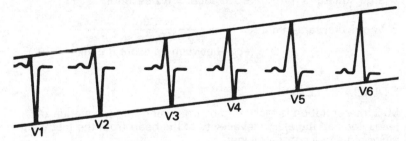

Clockwise or anticlockwise rotation is thus detected by these leads

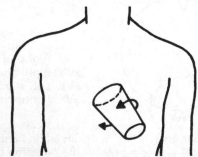

ARRHYTHMIAS

1. PREMATURE BEATS

Arise from ectopic focus in atrium, AV node or ventricle.
Usually followed by 'compensatory pause'

Supraventricular extrasystole
P is premature and may be bizarre

Nodal extrasystole
Essentially normal QRS but no preceding P

Ventricular extrasystole
Bizarre QRS with no preceding P

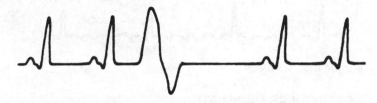

2. PAROXYSMAL ATRIAL TACHYCARDIA (PAT)

Normal QRS, but T waves altered by fusion with P waves

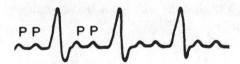

PAT with block (usually induced by digitalis)
Rapid regular P waves with slower QRS waves

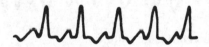

3. PAROXYSMAL VENTRICULAR TACHYCARDIA

QRS complexes are slurred and wide but fairly regular. P
waves often obscured

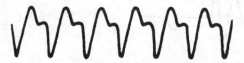

4. ATRIAL FIBRILLATION

Absent P waves and QRS complexes irregularly irregular

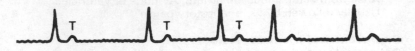

5. ATRIAL FLUTTER

P waves in 'sawtooth' pattern at 250–350/min and QRS complexes after every 2nd, 3rd or 4th P. The block may fluctuate rapidly, causing QRS to appear irregular

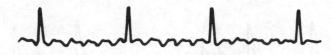

Flutter with 5:1 block

6. VENTRICULAR FIBRILLATION

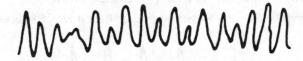

Rapid bizarre ventricular patterns

HEART BLOCK

BUNDLE-BRANCH BLOCK (BBB)

QRS exceeds 0.12 seconds with a notched complex

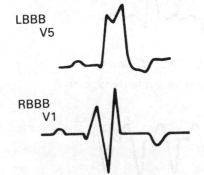

LBBB
V5

M-shaped wave in L chest leads
W-shaped wave in R chest leads

RBBB
V1

M-shaped wave in R chest leads
W-shaped wave in L chest leads

Mnemonic — WILLIAM MORROW
V1   V5
W — L — M = LBBB
M — R — W = RBBB

FIRST DEGREE BLOCK

PR interval exceeds 0.20 seconds but rhythm is normal

SECOND DEGREE BLOCK

QRS occurs only after every 2nd, 3rd or 4th P wave
P waves regular, but some obscured by T or QRS complexes

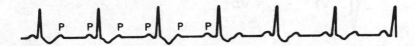

Wenkebach phenomenon (Mobitz type I)
PR interval progressively increases until a QRS is dropped, after
which PR shortens and the cycle is repeated

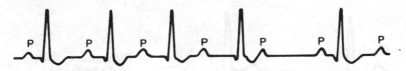

Mobitz type II
PR interval is constant but an occasional P wave is not followed by
a QRS complex

Third degree block (complete heart block)
P waves and QRS complexes occur completely independently of
each other. Ventricular rate is 25–50/min

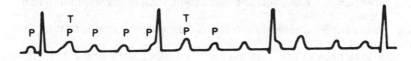

VENTRICULAR HYPERTROPHY
LVH

1. Tall R waves in left chest leads with deep S waves in right chest
   leads
   Sum of S in V1 and R in V5 exceeds 37 mm

2. May be LV 'strain' (ST depression and T inversion)
3. Left axis deviation
4. QRS may be slightly prolonged

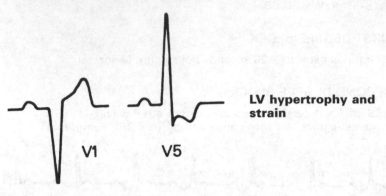

LV hypertrophy and strain

RVH

1. Tall R waves in right chest leads with S waves in left chest leads
2. R axis deviation

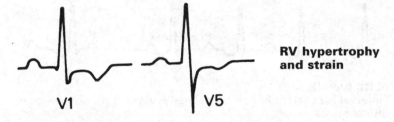

RV hypertrophy and strain

OTHER CAUSES OF ECG CHANGES

MYOCARDIAL INFARCTION

Characteristic changes are:
1. Transient ST elevation and persistent T wave inversion in leads facing the infarct
2. Transient ST depression in leads diametrically opposite the infarct
3. Appearance of Q waves exceeding 0.04 seconds and 2 mm deep. These occur later and persist

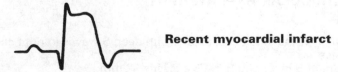

Recent myocardial infarct

Anterior infarct
Usually due to occlusion of the descending L coronary artery. The infarct faces leads I, aVL and the chest leads

Inferior (diaphragmatic) infarct
Due to occlusion of R coronary or circumflex artery. Faces leads II, III and aVF. Persistence of the acute infarction pattern for more than 6 months suggests ventricular aneurysm

MYOCARDIAL ISCHAEMIA WITHOUT INFARCTION
ST depression and symmetrical T wave inversion

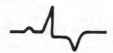

DIGITALIS

Also causes ST depression and T inversion but in a 'reversed tick' pattern

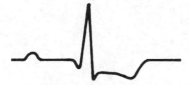

Digitalis also causes:
1. Bradycardia
2. Prolonged PR
3. Shortened QT
4. Any arrhythmia, especially bigemini or heart block

HYPOKALAEMIA

Prolongation of QT interval, ST depression and T wave flattening or inversion. Prominent U waves, which may fuse with the succeeding P

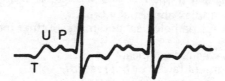

HYPERKALAEMIA

Small P waves with tall peaked T waves
QRS complex widens, and ventricular fibrillation may follow

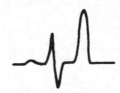

PERICARDITIS

Acute
Mexican saddle-shaped ST elevation in all the standard leads except aVR, and in most of the chest leads

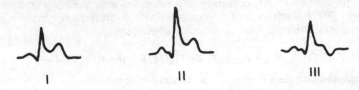

I   II   III

Chronic
ST becomes isoelectric and the T wave flattens and may invert

ACUTE PULMONARY EMBOLISM (classically 'S1, Q3, T3')

1. S wave in lead I
2. T wave inversion and Q wave in leads III and V1–V3
3. Transient RBBB
4. Right axis deviation

COR PULMONALE

1. Large pointed P waves
2. Changes of RV hypertrophy

HOW TO READ AN ECG

1. Identify the rhythm and rate
2. Are normal P waves present and what is the PR interval?
3. Is the cardiac axis normal?
4. Is the QRS complex abnormally broad?
   (LBBB is always pathological and makes further interpretation impossible)
5. Are the Q waves pathological?
6. Is the ST segment raised or depressed?
7. Are the T waves normal or inverted?

Further reading: *The ECG made easy*, J R Hampton, Churchill Livingstone, Edinburgh

4. Chest disease

LUNG VOLUMES

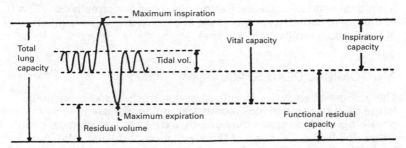

The resting expiratory level is the most constant reference point on the spirometer tracing

MINUTE VENTILATION

Product of tidal volume and number of respirations per minute

VITAL CAPACITY

Largest volume a subject can expire after a single maximal inspiration. Normal values increase with size of subject and decrease with age (about $4\frac{1}{2}$ litres in young adult male). Can be reduced in practically any lung or chest wall disease

FORCED VITAL CAPACITY (FVC)

The vital capacity when the expiration is performed as rapidly as possible

FEV_1

(Forced expiratory volume in one second) — volume expired during first second of FVC

Ratio $\dfrac{FEV_1}{FVC}$ should be 0.75 or more

The ratio is reduced in obstructive airway diseases (asthma, emphysema, bronchitis)

PEAK EXPIRATORY FLOW RATE (PEFR)

Maximum expiratory flow rate achieved during a forced expiration. A convenient way to detect a reduction in ventilatory function. Also useful for serial measurements in the same patient and for assessing response to bronchodilators

RESIDUAL VOLUME

Obtained by subtracting expiratory reserve volume from functional residual capacity. Residual volume is normally 20–25% of total lung capacity but increases in elderly, and in over-inflation of the lungs (emphysema, asthma)

ANATOMICAL DEAD SPACE

The volume of air in the mouth, pharynx, trachea and bronchi up to the terminal bronchioles (about 150 ml). In disease the physiological dead space may greatly exceed the anatomical dead space due to the disorders of the ventilation/perfusion ratio, but in health the two are identical

DIFFUSION DEFECTS

Carbon dioxide is about 20 times more diffusible than oxygen. In diffusion defects the *arterial* P_{O_2} is normal or slightly reduced at rest, but decreases markedly after exercise due to increased tissue uptake of O_2. Arterial P_{CO_2} is normal or even reduced at rest (due to hyperventilation) and tends to fall on exercise

DLCO is the transfer factor measured by carbon monoxide inhalation

VA is the alveolar volume measured by helium dilution

$$KCO, \text{ the gas transfer coefficient, } = \frac{DLCO}{VA}$$

CAUSES OF REDUCED DIFFUSING CAPACITY (TRANSFER FACTOR)

1. Alveolo-capillary block
    (i) Pulmonary oedema
    (ii) Pulmonary fibrosis
    (iii) Infiltrative lesions, e.g. sarcoidosis
2. Reduction in area available for diffusion
    (i) Emphysema
    (ii) Multiple pulmonary emboli
3. Haemorrhage into the alveoli (an artefact rather than a true reduction)

LUNG COMPLIANCE

A measure of lung elasticity. Compliance is reduced when the lungs are abnormally stiff due to pulmonary venous congestion or infiltrative or fibrotic lesions of the lungs

BLOOD-GAS ANALYSIS

These values must be related to the normal levels expected for the subject, e.g. baby, old man, pregnant woman

HYPOXIA

Oxygen deficiency at a specified site

HYPOXAEMIA

Oxygen deficiency in the blood. In arterial blood of normal resting adult:
Pco_2 is about 40 mmHg (4 to 6 kPa)
Po_2 is about 90 to 100 mmHg (12 to 15 kPa)

Causes of hypoxaemia
1. Cardio-respiratory disorders
    (i) Hypoventilation
    (ii) Abnormality of ventilation/perfusion (V/Q) ratio
    (iii) Impaired diffusion
    (iv) Venous to arterial shunt
2. Decreased Po_2 of inspired gas, e.g. high altitude
3. Reduction in active haemoglobin, e.g. carbon monoxide

   Type 1 respiratory failure, with $Pao_2 < 8$ kPa and $Paco_2 < 6.5$ kPa, occurs in asthma, LVF and pulmonary embolism
   Type 2 respiratory failure, with $Pao_2 < 8$ kPa and $Paco_2 > 6.5$ kPa, occurs in chronic bronchitis, CNS disease and impaired chest wall movement

HYPOVENTILATION

Reduction in lung ventilation sufficient to cause hypercapnia

Causes of hypoventilation
1. Respiratory centre depression, e.g. drugs, anoxia, central sleep apnoea
2. Neurological disease, e.g. polio, motor neurone disease
3. Respiratory muscle disease, e.g. dermatomyositis, Duchenne's muscular dystrophy
4. Limited chest movement, e.g. kyphoscoliosis, thoracoplasty for TB
5. Limited lung movement, e.g. pleural effusion, pneumothorax

6. Lung disease, e.g. collapse, pneumonia
7. Upper airway obstruction, e.g. obstructive sleep apnoea

DYSPNOEA

Subjective awareness of the need for an increased respiratory effort

KUSSMAUL'S BREATHING (AIR HUNGER)

Occurs in acidosis (uraemia, diabetes mellitus) due to stimulation of respiratory centre

CHEYNE–STOKES BREATHING

Amplitude of respiration progressively deepens to a maximum, then decreases to a period of apnoea. Due to diminished sensitivity of respiratory centre to CO_2. Occurs in left ventricular failure, central respiratory depression and in normal infants

OXYGEN THERAPY

In chronic hypoxia due to hypoventilation (e.g. chronic bronchitis) the arterial P_{CO_2} is raised and correction of the hypoxia by oxygen in high concentration may release the respiratory centre from its 'anoxic drive' and produce CO_2 narcosis. Low-concentration (24%) oxygen masks such as the Ventimask should be used, with serial blood gas analyses. If CO_2 continues to rise, respiratory stimulants or mechanical ventilation may be needed.

In hypoxia due to impaired gas exchange (e.g. pneumonia, pulmonary oedema) high concentration masks delivering 35–60% oxygen are required

DEFINITIONS OF COMMON PULMONARY DISEASE

CHRONIC BRONCHITIS

Chronic or recurrent increase in the volume of mucoid bronchial secretion sufficient to cause expectoration (usually daily cough with sputum for 3 months each year for at least 2 consecutive years). There is an obstructive element which is only partially reversible

EMPHYSEMA (defined histologically)

Is characterized by enlargement of the air spaces distal to the terminal bronchioles, with destruction of the alveolar walls

CHRONIC OBSTRUCTIVE AIRWAYS DISEASE (COAD)

This comprises chronic bronchitis and emphysema, which are often present simultaneously. Bronchiectasis is often misdiagnosed as bronchitis

ASTHMA

Is characterized by variable, often paroxysmal, dyspnoea due to widespread narrowing of the bronchioles. PEFR or FEV_1 is decreased, but at least 20% of the decrease must be reversible over a few minutes or days

Features of a *severe* asthma attack in an adult
1. Can't complete sentences in one breath
2. Respiratory rate exceeds 24/min
3. Pulse exceeds 110/min
4. PEFR less than 50% of predicted or previous best

Features of a *life-threatening* asthma attack
1. PEFR less than 33% of predicted or previous best
2. Silent chest, cyanosis or feeble respiratory effort
3. Bradycardia or hypotension
4. Exhaustion, confusion or coma
   If any of the above are present, measure the blood gases

Blood gas markers of a life-threatening attack
1. Normal or high $Paco_2$
2. Severe hypoxia, Pao_2 less than 8 kPa despite oxygen therapy
3. Low pH

HARMFUL EFFECTS OF CIGARETTE SMOKING

1. PHARMACOLOGICAL EFFECTS OF NICOTINE

   Rise in BP, tachycardia, increased platelet stickiness, etc.

2. PHARYNGEAL AND BRONCHIAL IRRITATION

   Bronchitis, post-op. pneumonia, etc.

3. CARCINOMA RISK INCREASED

   Bronchus, oesophagus, prostate, bladder

4. CARDIOVASCULAR DISEASE

   Myocardial ischaemia, Buerger's disease, 'strokes'

5. OSTEOPOROSIS RISK INCREASED

6. PASSIVE SMOKING EFFECTS
   (i) Effect on fetus due to smoking in pregnancy: restricted growth, increased perinatal mortality
   (ii) Effect on non-smokers: cough, asthma, angina

COMMON CAUSES OF CLUBBING

RESPIRATORY

1. Bronchial carcinoma
2. Chronic pulmonary suppuration, e.g. bronchiectasis, cystic fibrosis

CARDIOVASCULAR

1. Bacterial endocarditis
2. Cyanotic congenital heart disease

LESS COMMON CAUSES INCLUDE:

1. Asbestosis, especially with mesothelioma
2. Fibrosing alveolitis
3. Ulcerative colitis & Crohn's
4. Malabsorption
5. Cirrhosis
6. Graves' disease
7. Brachial arteriovenous fistula (unilateral)
8. Familial

HAEMOPTYSIS

COMMON CAUSES

Respiratory
1. Bronchial carcinoma
2. Pulmonary tuberculosis
3. Bronchitis
4. Bronchiectasis
5. Lung abscess

Cardiovascular
1. Pulmonary infarct
2. Mitral stenosis
3. Acute left ventricular failure

Less common causes include:
1. Pneumonia, especially pneumococcal
2. Collagen–vascular disease, especially polyarteritis nodosa

3. Idiopathic pulmonary haemosiderosis
4. Bleeding diathesis
5. Mycoses, e.g. aspergillosis
6. Foreign body
7. Hereditary haemorrhagic telangiectasia
8. Wegener's granulomatosis
9. Goodpasture's syndrome

Exclude spurious haemoptysis (nasal bleeding, etc.)

In many patients with a small haemoptysis and negative physical findings, no cause is ever found despite follow-up with serial chest X-rays

PNEUMONIA

Primary pneumonias are usually acquired in the community
　Secondary pneumonias occur when the lungs are already diseased

AETIOLOGICAL CLASSIFICATION

1. Infective
(i) *Bacterial*
  a. Strep. pneumoniae
  b. Mycoplasma pneumoniae
  c. Haemophilus influenzae
  d. Legionella pneumophila
  e. Chlamydia psittaci
  f. Staph. aureus (may be abscesses)
  g. Klebsiella pneumoniae (may cavitate)
  h. Mycobacteria (e.g. TB)
  Pneumonia may also be a feature of generalized bacterial infections, e.g. brucellosis, typhoid fever, plague
(ii) *Viral*
  a. Respiratory syncytial
  b. Influenza (usually secondary bacterial infection)
  c. Mumps (usually secondary bacterial infection)
  d. Cytomegalovirus
  e. URT viruses (adenovirus, rhinovirus, parainfluenza)
(iii) *Rickettsial*
  a. Typhus
  b. Q fever
(iv) *Yeasts and fungi*
  a. Candida
  b. Histoplasma
(v) *Protozoa and parasites*
  a. Pneumocystis carinii
  b. Toxoplasma
  c. Amoebae

2. Allergic

Collagen–vascular disease (esp. polyarteritis nodosa)
Stevens–Johnson syndrome (erythema multiforme)

3. Chemical agents

  (i) Irritant gases: NH_3, SO_2, Cl_2, oxides of nitrogen
 (ii) Irritant liquids: vomitus, lipoid pneumonia

4. Physical agents — irradiation

In discussing causes of pneumonia remember the possibility of
1. Opportunistic organisms in immune deficiency, especially AIDS
2. Pre-existing lung disease, e.g. bronchial carcinoma and bronchiectasis, especially if the pneumonia is recurrent or unresponsive
3. Inhalation pneumonia
    (i) Oral and pharyngeal sepsis and sinusitis
   (ii) Oesophageal obstruction and pharyngeal pouch
  (iii) Alcoholic debauch, drowning or anaesthesia
  (iv) Laryngeal cancer
   (v) Tracheo-oesophageal fistula
  (vi) Inadequate gag reflex
4. Predisposing systemic disease such as diabetes, cirrhosis, alcoholism or agranulocytosis
5. Foreign body not seen on X-ray (e.g. peanut)

COMPLICATIONS OF PNEUMOCOCCAL LOBAR PNEUMONIA

1. Pleurisy with effusion, or serous pericarditis
2. Empyema or pericardial suppuration
3. Endocarditis, meningitis (not to be confused with meningismus, in which CSF is normal) or cerebral abscess
4. Delayed resolution
5. Nonspecific complications
    (i) Herpes labialis
   (ii) Septicaemia (may be 'shock')
  (iii) Cardiac failure
  (iv) Cardiac arrhythmia
   (v) Deep vein thrombosis

CAUSES OF EMPYEMA

1. Pneumonia, especially lobar, or secondary to bronchial Ca
2. Lung abscess
3. Subphrenic abscess
4. Mediastinal sepsis
5. Chest wound or surgery
6. TB

CAUSES OF PULMONARY COLLAPSE

1. ABSORPTION COLLAPSE

   Due to complete bronchial obstruction
   - (i) Intraluminal, e.g. foreign body, mucus or clot
   - (ii) Mural, e.g. bronchial carcinoma or adenoma
   - (iii) Extramural, e.g. peribronchial lymphadenopathy or aortic aneurysm

2. PNEUMOTHORAX OR PLEURAL EFFUSION

   Remember that in absorption collapse the mediastinum shifts to the affected side, but in collapse due to air or fluid in the pleural space the mediastinum may shift to the opposite side

CAUSES OF PLEURAL EFFUSION

TRANSUDATE

(Less than 30 g protein/litre. Implies a systemic cause)
1. Cardiac failure
2. Nephrotic syndrome
3. Hepatic failure

EXUDATE

(More than 30 g protein/litre. Implies a local cause)
1. **P**ulmonary emboli
2. **R**heumatoid disease
3. **I**nfections (pneumonia, TB)
4. **S**LE and other collagen–vascular diseases
5. **M**alignancy (bronchial Ca, secondary Ca, Hodgkin's, mesothelioma)
6. **S**ubphrenic abscess
   Mnemonic: PRISMS

CAUSES OF PNEUMOTHORAX

1. Traumatic
2. Iatrogenic, e.g. thoracentesis or surgery
3. Spontaneous
   - (i) Subpleural bulla
   - (ii) Emphysema
   - (iii) Asthma
   - (iv) TB
   - (v) Lung abscess
   - (vi) Pneumoconiosis

CAUSES OF ACUTE PULMONARY OEDEMA

1. Left heart failure
   (i) Atrial, e.g. mitral stenosis
   (ii) Ventricular, e.g. hypertension or myocardial infarct
2. Overload of i.v. fluid
3. Inhalation of irritant gas, e.g. chlorine, dense smoke
4. Fulminating viral or bacterial pneumonia
5. Fat emboli
6. Neurogenic (rare)
   e.g. Head injury or cerebro-vascular accident

CAUSES OF INTERSTITIAL LUNG DISEASE

1. Cryptogenic fibrosing alveolitis
2. Sarcoidosis
3. Extrinsic allergic alveolitis
4. Asbestosis, pneumoconiosis or silicosis
5. Drugs or irradiation
6. Pulmonary eosinophilia
7. Collagen–vascular disease

BRONCHIECTASIS

Permanent dilatation of the bronchi, usually accompanied by recurrent bronchial suppuration

PATHOGENESIS

Animal experiments suggest that proximal narrowing of the airways and distal infection are both important

CAUSES

1. Infection
   (i)   Bronchiolitis of infancy
   (ii) Measles or pertussis in children
   (iii) Post broncho-pneumonic collapse in adults
   (iv) Commonly in post-primary TB
2. Bronchial stenosis or occlusion
   (i)   Adenoma or carcinoma
   (ii) Foreign body or asthma casts
   (iii) Lymphadenopathy
3. Pulmonary aspergillosis
4. Cystic fibrosis
5. Hypogammaglobulinaemia
6. Ciliary dysfunction (e.g. Kartagener's syndrome)
7. Many cases are idiopathic

CLINICAL FEATURES

1. Classical symptom — cough with copious purulent sputum, especially on changing posture
2. Classical sign — localized persistent coarse crepitations
3. May be asymptomatic
4. Malaise, intermittent fever, halitosis
5. Weight loss or 'failure to thrive'
6. Dyspnoea, cyanosis or clubbing
7. Haemoptysis

TYPES OF CA BRONCHUS

1. **S**quamous (35%)
2. **O**at cell (small cell) (25%)
3. **L**arge cell (20%)
4. **A**denocarcinoma (20%)
   Mnemonic: SOLA

COMPLICATIONS OF CA BRONCHUS

LOCAL EFFECTS

1. Bronchial obstruction: collapse, consolidation, abscess
2. Malignant pleural effusion
3. Erosion of large vessel
4. Superior vena caval obstruction
5. Direct spread to chest wall, brachial plexus (Pancoast's)
6. **H**orner's syndrome from cervical sympathetic compression
   Hoarseness from recurrent laryngeal nerve compression
   High diaphragm from phrenic nerve involvement

METASTASES

Especially hilar nodes, liver, brain, bone, adrenals

NON-METASTATIC EXTRA-PULMONARY EFFECTS

1. Cachexia and anaemia
2. Clubbing (hypertrophic pulmonary osteoarthropathy)
3. Endocrine
    (i) Gynaecomastia
   (ii) Inappropriate ADH → hyponatraemia (often small cell)
   (iii) Inappropriate PTH → hypercalcaemia (often squamous)
   (iv) Inappropriate ACTH → pigmentation, hypokalaemia, alkalosis (often small cell)
4. Dermatological
   Pigmentation, pruritus, etc. (see page 156)
5. Neuropathy or myopathy (incl. dermatomyositis and Eaton–Lambert syndrome)

TUBERCULOSIS

PRIMARY TB

Occurs in subjects never previously exposed to TB
'Primary complex' = Ghon focus + regional lymphadenopathy
Abdominal primary TB and tuberculous cervical lymphadenitis are
now uncommon in the United Kingdom, except in the immigrant
population

PULMONARY PRIMARY TB

Usually heals spontaneously

Complications
1. Local spread in lung
2. Cavitation
3. Pleural effusion (may develop before positive Mantoux)
4. Rupture of caseous node into bronchus causing widespread
   bronchopneumonia
5. Segmental collapse due to bronchial compression by nodes
6. 'Middle lobe syndrome', i.e. bronchiectasis in later life due to
   bronchial compression by nodes
7. Haematogenous metastasis
     (i)   Bone
    (ii)   Kidney
   (iii)   Epididymis or Fallopian tubes
    (iv)   Meninges
8. Miliary TB

POST-PRIMARY TB

Reinfection or recrudescence of primary lesion. Usually
pulmonary, but may be miliary or atypical in the old or
immunosuppressed

PULMONARY TB

Complications
1. Caseation ('cold abscess')
2. Bronchogenic spread in lungs
3. Pleurisy
4. Effusion or TB empyema
5. Haemoptysis, may be massive
6. Tension cavity due to valvular obstruction
7. Tuberculoma of lungs
8. Haematogenous metastasis or miliary TB
9. Chronic pulmonary fibrosis and compensatory emphysema
   (especially in miners)

10. TB tracheitis, laryngitis or stomatitis due to expectoration of mycobacteria
11. Swallowed sputum may cause intestinal TB (usually in lymphoid patches)
12. Amyloidosis

COMMON PRESENTATIONS OF PULMONARY TB

1. Asymptomatic (screening CXR)
2. Persistent cough
3. Tiredness, malaise, recurrent coryza, weight loss or fever
4. Pneumonia
5. Haemoptysis
6. Dyspepsia

Note increased incidence in immigrants, elderly, immunosuppressed, diabetic and after gastrectomy for peptic ulcer

SARCOIDOSIS

Definition: a multisystem granulomatous disease (of unknown origin), in which the granulomas consist of well-formed, sharply demarcated collections of epithelioid cells, with little or no caseation, and little cellular reaction around them

CLINICAL FEATURES OF SARCOIDOSIS

1. Pulmonary:
   Bilateral hilar lymphadenopathy (BHL)
   ↓
   BHL + pre-fibrotic pulmonary infiltration
   ↓
   Either resolution or pulmonary fibrosis
2. Constitutional symptoms, febrile arthralgia
3. Superficial lymphadenopathy
4. Skin lesions — erythema nodosum, lupus pernio, infiltrated plaques, nodules, infiltrates in scars
5. Ocular lesions — uveitis, conjunctival infiltrates, etc.
6. Parotid, lacrimal gland lesions
7. Neurological lesions
   (i) Neuropathy, especially facial nerve
   (ii) Meningeal infiltration and local CNS deposits
8. Liver, spleen or cardiac infiltration
9. Bone involvement, especially phalangeal cysts
10. Hypercalcaemia ± nephrocalcinosis and calculi

PHYSICAL SIGNS IN LUNG DISEASE

	Chest wall movement	Mediastinum and trachea	Tactile vocal fremitus	Percussion note	Breath sounds	Added sounds
Large pleural effusion	Decreased on affected side	Shift to opposite side	Absent	Stony dull	Absent. May be bronchial (± whispering pectoriloquy) above fluid level	Absent. May be pleural rub above fluid
Consolidation	Decreased on affected side	Central	Increased	Dull	Bronchial	Fine or medium crackles
Massive collapse	Decreased on affected side	Shift to affected side	Absent	Dull	Decreased	Absent
Fibrosis	Local flattening with decreased movement	Shift to affected side	Increased	Dull	Bronchial	May be coarse crepitations
Large pneumothorax	Decreased on affected side	Shift to opposite side	Decreased	Increased	Decreased	Absent unless bowel sounds are transmitted
Emphysema	Decreased bilateral ('barrel chest')	Central (except in unilateral emphysema)	Decreased	Increased	Decreased	Absent
Bronchitis	Decreased bilaterally ('barrel chest')	Central	Normal or decreased	Increased	Decreased	Wheezes and crackles

5. Chest X-rays

HOW TO LOOK AT A CHEST X-RAY

1. Name, age of patient, date of X-ray
2. Is it a PA film (usual) or an AP film? (implying the patient was too ill to stand up for the film, and thus preventing assessment of heart size)
3. Is the film well orientated and correctly penetrated?
4. **The lungs and hila**
   Count the visible **R**ibs to assess the size of the lungs
   Look at the lung fields for any **A**symmetry
   Is the **T**rachea displaced?
   Are there any abnormalities in the lung **F**ields?
   Are the **A**pices clear? (check for TB or small pneumothorax)
   Are the **C**osto-phrenic angles blunted?
   Are the hila **E**nlarged?
   Mnemonic: RATFACE
5. **The heart**
   Is it enlarged and is its outline normal?
6. **The ribs and spine**
   Look for fractures, metastases, rib notches, etc.
7. **Any other shadows?**
   Tracheostomy, central line, prosthetic heart valves, ECG monitor wires, jewellery, pyjama buttons, etc.
8. **Any gas outside the chest?**
   Surgical emphysema, gas under R diaphragm, etc.

CAUSES OF WHOLE LUNG OPACITY

1. Consolidation of L lung   **2. Massive L pleural effusion**

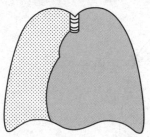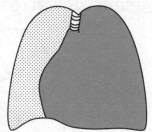

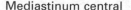

Mediastinum central   Mediastinum and trachea move to R

3. Collapse of entire L lung

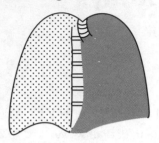

Features
1. Trachea pulled to L
2. R heart border not seen
3. L diaphragm obscured
4. R lung hypertranslucent

COLLAPSE OF R UPPER LOBE

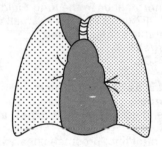

Features
1. Dense wedge against superior mediastinum
2. R hilar vessels drawn up, and widely spaced
3. R lower and middle lobes hypertranslucent
4. Trachea and aortic knob pulled to R

COLLAPSE OF L LOWER LOBE

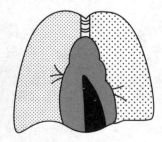

Features
1. Dense wedge in heart shadow and diaphragm behind L side of heart obscured
2. L hilar vessels pulled down and widely spaced
3. L upper lobe hypertranslucent

R PLEURAL EFFUSION

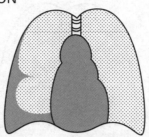

Note fluid in horizontal fissure

SMALL L PNEUMOTHORAX

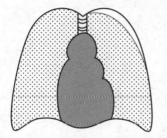

R HYDROPNEUMOTHORAX

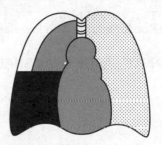

Usually traumatic
(including pleural aspiration)

PULMONARY OEDEMA

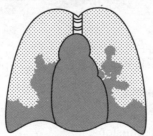

Features
1. 'Bats-wing' shadows — ill defined and confluent, spreading out from hila

2. Generalized lower-zone haze
3. Upper lobe diversion of blood
4. Kerley B lines
5. Enlarged heart

EMPHYSEMA

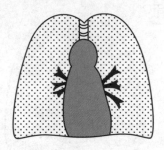

Features
1. Hypertranslucent lung fields
2. Main pulmonary vessels are large, but peripheral vessels are thin
3. Thin vertical heart
4. Horizontal ribs with low flat diaphragm

SINGLE LARGE OVAL SHADOW

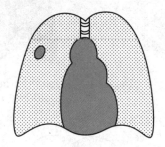

Common causes
1. Bronchial cancer
2. Metastatic deposit, e.g. breast cancer, hypernephroma

Less common causes
3. TB (may be calcified)
4. Abscess
5. Encysted pleural effusion
6. Cyst, e.g. hydatid
7. Adenoma, fibroma or hamartoma
8. AV aneurysm

MULTIPLE CIRCULAR SHADOWS

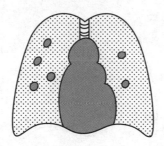

Causes
1. Metastatic malignancy
2. Hydatid cysts
3. Caplan's syndrome (rheumatoid arthritis with pneumoconiosis)
4. Multiple lung abscesses
5. Wegener's granulomatosis

WIDESPREAD SHADOWING

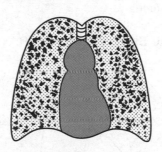

Causes include
1. Miliary TB
2. Pulmonary oedema
3. Bronchopneumonia
4. Pneumoconiosis or haemosiderosis
5. Sarcoidosis
6. Systemic sclerosis
7. Fibrosing alveolitis and rheumatoid lung
8. Hypersensitivity, e.g. allergic alveolitis ('farmer's lung', etc.)
9. Neoplasm:
   Miliary Ca metastases
   Lymphangitis carcinomatosa
   Alveolar cell carcinoma
10. Post-viral pneumonia with miliary calcification (esp. varicella)

BILATERAL HILAR LYMPHADENOPATHY

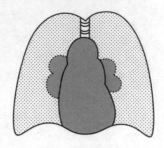

Causes include
1. Sarcoidosis
2. Lymphocytic leukaemia
3. Lymphoma
4. Carcinoma metastases
5. Primary tuberculosis
6. Acute infections, e.g. infectious mononucleosis or whooping-cough

If unilateral, examine lung fields carefully for bronchial carcinoma or Ghon focus

NORMAL CARDIAC SHADOW IN PA X-RAY

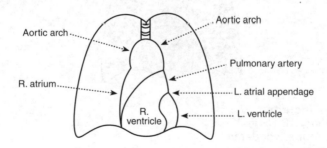

Transverse diameter of heart does not normally exceed 50% of chest width

SYSTEMIC HYPERTENSION

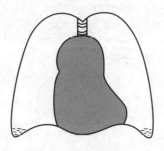

Features
1. Aortic unfolding
2. LV hypertrophy
3. Kerley B lines (horizontal lines in costophrenic angles due to dilated subpleural lymphatics) if LV failure develops

MITRAL STENOSIS

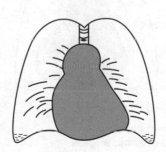

Features
1. Straight L heart border and convex R border
2. Increased pulmonary vascular shadows
3. Kerley B lines

COARCTATION OF AORTA

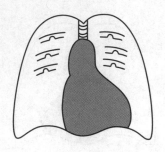

Features
1. LV hypertrophy
2. Small aortic arch
3. Rib notching

PERICARDIAL EFFUSION

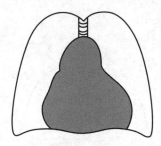

Features
1. Large rounded heart shadow
2. Note sharp cardio-phrenic angles

   Distinction from dilated heart may be very difficult

6. Gastroenterology

CAUSES OF ATROPHIC GLOSSITIS *(SMOOTH RED TONGUE)*

1. Antibiotics
2. Anaemia due to deficiency of Fe, B_{12} or folate
3. Vitamin deficiency (riboflavin or nicotinic acid)

CAUSES OF DYSPHAGIA

1. LESIONS OF MOUTH OR PHARYNX

    (i) Stomatitis or glossitis
    (ii) Tonsillitis
    (iii) Quinsy, retropharyngeal abscess
    (iv) Lymphoma of tonsil

2. FOREIGN BODY IN PHARYNX OR OESOPHAGUS

3. INTRINSIC DISEASE OF PHARYNX OR OESOPHAGUS

    (i) Plummer–Vinson syndrome — iron deficiency, glossitis, pharyngeal web and koilonychia
    (ii) Pharyngeal pouch
    (iii) Inflammation, stricture or neoplasm of oesophagus
    (iv) Systemic sclerosis
    (v) Oesophageal achalasia

4. EXTRINSIC COMPRESSION

    (i) Tumours in neck
    (ii) Mediastinal tumour, e.g. retrosternal goitre, lymph nodes
    (iii) Bronchial cancer
    (iv) Aortic aneurysm

5. CNS LESIONS

    (i) Bulbar or pseudo-bulbar palsy
    (ii) Myasthenia gravis
    (iii) Congenital muscular incoordination

COMMON CAUSES OF SEVERE UPPER GI BLEEDING

1. Duodenal ulcer
2. Oesophageal varices
3. Erosive gastritis (e.g. due to aspirin or NSAID)
4. Gastric ulcer (may be malignant)
5. Erosive oesophagitis (e.g. hiatus hernia)

COMMON CAUSES OF SEVERE LOWER GI BLEEDING

1. Colonic diverticular disease
2. Carcinoma of rectum or colon
3. Benign rectal polyps
4. Haemorrhoids or anal fissure
5. Colonic angiodysplasia
6. Ulcerative colitis or Crohn's disease
7. Rectal trauma, including biopsy
8. Hookworm (in tropics)

N.B. Hiatus hernia, colonic diverticulosis and haemorrhoids are common. Massive blood loss should not be attributed to them unless the source of bleeding can be seen, or more serious pathology can be excluded

MEDICAL CAUSES OF ACUTE ABDOMINAL PAIN

1. Food poisoning or dietary indiscretion
2. Peptic ulcer, gastritis, oesophagitis
3. Biliary colic or cholecystitis
4. Pancreatitis
5. Hepatic congestion (hepatitis, cardiac failure)
6. Renal colic, pyelonephritis, cystitis, acute urinary retention
7. Diverticulitis, ulcerative colitis, Crohn's disease
8. Mesenteric adenitis (children)
9. Constipation
10. Mesenteric ischaemia (atheroma, embolism, polyarteritis nodosa)
11. Aortic dissection
12. Gynaecological, e.g.
     Mittelschmerz (ovulation)
     Dysmenorrhoea
     Salpingitis
     Threatened abortion
13. Pain referred from spine or chest (e.g. myocardial infarct)

N.B. Pain in the abdomen which lasts for more than 6 hours without remission is likely to be surgical
Rarer causes of acute abdominal pain include: acute intermittent porphyria, herpes zoster, diabetes mellitus (gastric dilatation),

sickle-cell crisis, lead poisoning, hereditary angio-oedema, Henoch–Schönlein purpura, etc.

PEPTIC ULCERS

DIFFERENCES BETWEEN GASTRIC AND DUODENAL ULCERS

	Gastric	Duodenal
Site	Usually middle 2/3 of lesser curve	Usually duodenal bulb
Gastric acid	Low or normal	Hyperchlorhydria
Pain	After meals	Relieved by meals May occur at about 2 a.m.
Vomiting	Common	Uncommon
Social class	Commoner in lower social classes	Equal prevalence
Pathology	May be benign or malignant	Virtually never malignant
Helicobacter pylori	70%	90%

FACTORS SUGGESTING A GASTRIC ULCER IS MALIGNANT

Symptoms
1. Anorexia and weight loss
2. Epigastric pain not related to food
3. Dysphagia

   N.B. The pain of both benign and malignant ulcers may be relieved by H_2-blockers

Signs
1. Epigastric mass
2. Metastases. Look especially for
   (i) Large irregular liver
   (ii) Supraclavicular nodes (Virchow's)
   (iii) Deep vein thrombosis of leg
   (iv) Ascites
   (v) Krukenberg tumour of ovary (felt PR)

Barium meal
1. Filling defect and failure of peristalsis in a site other than middle 2/3 of lesser curve
2. Very large ulcer anywhere in the stomach
3. Leather-bottle stomach

If in doubt gastroscopy (with biopsy) and gastric cytology should be performed

COMPLICATIONS OF PEPTIC ULCER

1. Bleeding
2. Penetration, e.g. into pancreas, liver or retroperitoneal space
3. Perforation
4. Obstruction
   - (i) Oedema and spasm — reversible
   - (ii) Cicatricial stenosis — irreversible
5. 'Milk–alkali syndrome' — alkalosis and calcinosis, due to excessive ingestion of milk, alkali and calcium salts

MALABSORPTION

CAUSES

1. **Inadequate digestion**
   - (i) Gastric or intestinal resection
   - (ii) Hepatic or biliary tract obstruction
   - (iii) Pancreatic insufficiency (especially cystic fibrosis)

2. **Parasites or change in intestinal flora**
   - (i) Tapeworms or Giardiasis
   - (ii) Blind-loop syndromes

3. **Tropical sprue**

4. **Intestinal hurry or fistulae**

5. **Coeliac disease**
   AIDS and erythroderma can also cause partial villous atrophy

6. **Intestinal infiltration**
   - (i) TB
   - (ii) Lymphoma or leukaemia
   - (iii) Systemic sclerosis
   - (iv) Intestinal lipodystrophy (Whipple's disease)

7. **Enzyme defects**
   - (i) Lactase deficiency
   - (ii) Hartnup disease

8. **Chronic intestinal ischaemia,** e.g. mesenteric atheroma

   N.B. The fat-soluble vitamins are D A K E

CLINICAL FEATURES OF COELIAC DISEASE IN ADULT
1. Loose stools which may or may not be bulky, pale and foul-smelling
2. Weight loss (fat and protein deficiency)
3. Oedema (protein deficiency)
4. Flatulence with distended abdomen (impaired disaccharide hydrolysis)
5. Hypochromic anaemia (Fe deficiency)
6. Macrocytic anaemia (folate or B_{12} deficiency)
7. Peripheral neuritis (B-complex deficiency)
8. Glossitis and stomatitis (B-complex deficiency)
9. Osteomalacia (Ca and vitamin D deficiency)
10. Paraesthesiae, tetany (Ca or Mg deficiency)
11. Haemorrhage (vitamin K deficiency)
12. Muscle flaccidity, arrhythmias (potassium deficiency)
13. Weakness and hypotension (water and electrolyte deficiency)
14. Clubbing
15. Dermatitis herpetiformis is strongly associated

AIDS AND THE GI TRACT

1. INFECTIONS ASSOCIATED WITH ANAL INTERCOURSE

   e.g. anal warts, herpes simplex, hepatitis A and B, etc.

2. OPPORTUNISTIC INFECTIONS

   e.g. candida, cryptosporidiosis, cytomegalovirus, mycobacteria

3. KAPOSI'S SARCOMA

4. LYMPHOMA

   May involve CNS, marrow or gut

5. PARTIAL VILLOUS ATROPHY WITH MALABSORPTION

CAUSES OF ASCITES

1. Carcinoma, especially ovarian or alimentary with peritoneal metastases
2. Cirrhosis
3. Hypoalbuminaemia, e.g. nephrotic syndrome
4. Constrictive pericarditis, congestive heart failure
5. Thrombosis or obstruction of inferior vena cava
6. Tuberculous peritonitis
7. Peritonitis in late stages
8. Chylous ascites due to lymphatic obstruction

CAUSES OF OBSTRUCTION OF THE SMALL INTESTINE

The commonest causes are adhesions secondary to operation and bowel incarceration in an internal or external hernia

MECHANICAL

1. Compression from without:
    (i) Adhesions
    (ii) Fibrous bands
    (iii) Tumours, especially of female pelvic organs
    (iv) Hernia
2. Compression from within the bowel wall:
    (i) Congenital atresia
    (ii) Acquired:
        Inflammatory
        Neoplastic
        Traumatic
3. Obstruction inside the lumen:
    (i) Gallstones
    (ii) Faecal impaction
    (iii) Meconium ileus
    (iv) Foreign bodies
    (v) Worms
4. Volvulus
5. Intussusception

PARALYTIC ILEUS (no colicky pain or bowel sounds)

1. Abdominal surgery
2. Peritonitis
3. Acute systemic illness, e.g. pneumonia
4. Painful lumbar conditions, e.g.
    renal colic
    retroperitoneal haematoma
5. Mesenteric ischaemia
6. Drugs, e.g. ganglion-blockers
7. Hypokalaemia
8. Hypothyroidism

DIVERTICULITIS

CLINICAL FEATURES

1. Usually middle-aged or elderly
2. Recurrent bouts of colicky abdominal pain
3. Nausea and vomiting
4. May be either constipation or diarrhoea
5. Tenderness in L iliac fossa, sometimes with a mass

COMPLICATIONS

1. Obstruction due to stricture
2. Perforation
3. Abscess
4. Fistula into bladder or vagina

BARIUM ENEMA

1. Diverticula may or may not be seen
2. Segmental spasm and irritability of the affected colon (usually sigmoid)
3. Chronic fibrotic deformity

ULCERATIVE COLITIS

CLINICAL FEATURES

1. Commonly presents in 3rd or 4th decade
2. Malaise, weakness, weight loss, pyrexia
3. Chronic diarrhoea, with blood and mucus, which is often severe
4. Pain in L iliac fossa, and rectal tenesmus

COMPLICATIONS

1. Perforation
2. Perianal abscess
3. Acute 'toxic dilatation'
4. Severe haemorrhage
5. Hypokalaemia, hypoproteinaemia, dehydration
6. Skin lesions:
    (i) Pyoderma gangrenosum
    (ii) Aphthous ulcers
    (iii) Erythema nodosum
    (iv) Clubbing
7. Diffuse liver disease and sclerosing cholangitis
8. Arthritis and uveitis
9. Amyloidosis after chronic abscesses
10. Carcinoma of colon

BARIUM ENEMA

1. Loss of haustration
2. Straight, narrow, inelastic colon
3. May be 'spicules' due to tiny ulcer craters
4. May be filling defects due to 'pseudopolyps'

   N.B. Abnormalities are usually continuous (no 'skip' lesions), and start at the rectum, affecting a variable length of the large bowel

CROHN'S DISEASE (REGIONAL ILEITIS)

CLINICAL FEATURES

1. Usually young adults
2. Malaise, weakness, weight loss, pyrexia
3. Intermittent colicky pain in R iliac fossa
4. Mild or moderate diarrhoea
5. Tenderness in R iliac fossa, sometimes with a fixed mass

COMPLICATIONS

1. Obstruction due to stricture
2. Perforation
3. Abscess
4. Fistula into anus, bladder or abdominal wall
5. Fissure-in-ano
6. Malabsorption (especially B_{12})
7. Proctocolitis
8. Erythema nodosum
9. Clubbing

BA STUDIES (may need both meal and enema)

1. Luminal narrowing of ileum (Kantor's 'string sign')
2. Distorted mucosal pattern
3. 'Skip' lesions

The correlation between radiological appearance and disease activity is often poor

FEATURES DISTINGUISHING CROHN'S AND ULCERATIVE COLITIS

	Crohn's	Ulcerative colitis
Granulomas	Present	Absent
Inflammation	Transmural	Confined to mucosa
Goblet cells	Normal number	Decreased
Crypt abscesses	Unusual	Common
Fistulae	Common	Uncommon
Skip lesions	Present	Absent
Terminal ileum	Usually involved	Rarely involved
Rectal involvement	Unusual	Almost invariable

CAUSES OF HEPATOMEGALY

1. Hepatic congestion, e.g. cardiac failure, hepatic vein thrombosis. The liver is pulsatile in severe tricuspid regurgitation

2. Neoplasm
    (i) Metastases
    (ii) Lymphoma
    (iii) Hepatoma
3. Myeloproliferative disease, e.g. leukaemia, myelofibrosis
4. Infective
    (i) Viral, e.g. hepatitis (q.v.)
    (ii) Bacterial, e.g. Weil's disease
    (iii) Protozoal, e.g. amoebic abscess
    (iv) Parasitic, e.g. hydatid cyst
5. Biliary obstruction, e.g. Ca pancreas
6. Fatty infiltration or early cirrhosis
7. Storage disorders, e.g. amyloidosis, Gaucher's

CAUSES OF A HARD KNOBBLY LIVER

1. Cancer metastases
2. Cirrhosis with hepatoma
3. Polycystic liver
4. Hydatid cysts

CAUSES OF HEPATO-SPLENOMEGALY

1. Infection, e.g. infectious mononucleosis
2. Myeloproliferative disease
3. Lymphoma
4. Storage diseases, e.g. amyloidosis, Gaucher's

CIRRHOSIS

Cirrhosis is characterized by hepatic parenchymal damage with fibrosis and nodular regeneration throughout the liver, accompanied by distortion of the normal lobular pattern

CAUSES OF CIRRHOSIS

1. Cryptogenic (idiopathic)
2. Alcoholism
3. Viral hepatitis (especially hepatitis B or C)
4. 'Autoimmune' liver disease
    (i) Primary biliary cirrhosis (antimitochondrial Ab in 95%)
    (ii) Chronic active hepatitis (smooth muscle Ab in 66%)
5. Haemochromatosis (primary or secondary)
6. Hepato-lenticular degeneration (Wilson's)
7. Hepatotoxins, e.g. methotrexate, carbon tetrachloride

CLINICAL FEATURES OF CIRRHOSIS

Features of hepatic failure
1. Firm hepatomegaly in the early stages
2. Low grade fever
3. Skin changes:
   (i) Jaundice in later stages
   (ii) 'Spiders'
   (iii) Palmar erythema
   (iv) Leuconychia (white nails)
4. Bleeding tendency (decreased coagulation factors)
5. Fatigue, weight loss, dyspepsia
6. Foetor hepaticus
7. Encephalopathy:
   (i) Lethargy
   (ii) Slow, slurred speech
   (iii) Flapping tremor
   (iv) Dementia
   (v) Precoma progressing to delirium and coma
8. Water retention:
   (i) Oedema
   (ii) Hyponatraemia

Features of portal hypertension
1. Splenomegaly, often with pancytopenia (hypersplenism)
2. GI bleeding from oesophageal varices
3. Ascites (low plasma albumin is also necessary)

Other features
1. Clubbing
2. Hyperkinetic circulation
3. Sexual changes:
   Females: erratic menstruation and breast atrophy
   Males: gynaecomastia, testicular atrophy and scanty body hair
4. Parotid enlargement ⎫
5. Dupuytren's contracture ⎭ in alcoholics
6. Susceptibility to infections

JAUNDICE

Jaundice (icterus) is due to hyperbilirubinaemia. It involves the sclerae, unlike the yellow pigmentation due to mepacrine or carotenaemia

CAUSES

Pre-hepatic
1. Haemolysis
2. Ineffective erythropoiesis

Hepatic

(a) Impaired conjugation
    (i) Hepatitis (viral or drug-induced)
    (ii) Gilbert's syndrome
(b) Impaired excretion
    (i) Hepatitis
    (ii) Methyltestosterone (dose-related)
    (iii) Chlorpromazine (hypersensitivity)
(c) Intra-hepatic obstruction
    (i) Hepatitis
    (ii) Cirrhosis
    (iii) Tumour

Post-hepatic

  (i) Stone in common bile duct (CBD)
  (ii) Carcinoma of head of pancreas or biliary tract
 (iii) Pressure on CBD from lymph nodes
 (iv) Stricture of CBD (post-operative or post-inflammatory)
  (v) Developmental anomalies (rare)

SUMMARY OF BLOOD CHANGES

	Obstructive	Hepatocellular failure with no obstruction	Haemolytic
Hyperbilirubinaemia	Conjugated	Unconjugated	Unconjugated
Alkaline phosphatase	Marked increase	Normal or increased	Slightly increased
Aspartate transaminase	Normal or slight increase	Increased	Normal

SUMMARY OF URINARY AND FAECAL BILE PIGMENT CHANGES

	Obstructive	Hepatocellular failure with no obstruction	Haemolytic
Urinary bilirubin	Increased	Normal or increased	Normal
Urinary urobilinogen	Decreased	Normal or increased	Increased
Faecal stercobilinogen	Decreased	Normal	Increased

VIRAL HEPATITIS

CAUSES

1. Hepatitis A — an enterovirus spread by the oral–faecal route. Does not cause chronic hepatitis

2. Hepatitis B (Australia Ag) — spread by blood or sexual intercourse. Worse prognosis if superinfected with hepatitis D
3. Hepatitis C — spread by blood or sexual intercourse
4. Hepatitis E — spread by the oral–faecal route. Dangerous in pregnancy
5. Cytomegalovirus
6. Infectious mononucleosis

COMPLICATIONS OF GALLSTONES
COMMON

1. Biliary colic
2. Cholecystitis or cholangitis
3. Obstructed neck of gallbladder
4. Pancreatitis

RARE

1. Gallstone ileus
2. Gallbladder perforation
3. Gallbladder cancer

CAUSES OF ACUTE PANCREATITIS

1. Biliary tract disease, including gallstones
2. Alcohol
3. Idiopathic
4. Metabolic, e.g. hyperparathyroidism, hypercalcaemia
5. Trauma, including surgery
6. Viral, e.g. mumps

CAUSES OF CHRONIC PANCREATITIS

1. Alcoholism
2. Malnutrition
3. Cystic fibrosis
4. Familial

7. Haematology

ANAEMIA (HB < 13.5 G/DL IN MALES, < 11.5 G/DL IN FEMALES)

CAUSES OF ANAEMIA

Deficient RBC production
1. Deficiency of:
    (i) Fe
    (ii) B_{12} or folic acid
    (iii) Vitamin C
    (iv) Protein
2. Aplastic anaemia (p. 79)
3. Marrow infiltration:
    (i) Leukaemia
    (ii) Lymphoma, e.g. Hodgkin's
    (iii) Myeloma
    (iv) Myelosclerosis
    (v) Metastatic carcinoma
4. 'Symptomatic' (anaemia of chronic disease)
    (i) Chronic infection
    (ii) Uraemia
    (iii) Liver disease
    (iv) Hypothyroidism
    (v) Hypopituitarism
    (vi) Malignancy
    (vii) Collagen–vascular disease, e.g. SLE, rheumatoid disease

Loss or destruction of RBCs
1. Haemorrhage
2. Haemolysis (p. 77)
3. Hypersplenism

SOME RBC ABNORMALITIES SEEN IN A BLOOD FILM

SIZE

Anisocytosis
Variation in size, due to anaemia

Macrocytosis
Seen in a film as increased diameter of RBCs, but defined as an increase in mean corpuscular *volume*

Microcytosis
Defined as a decrease in mean corpuscular *volume*

SHAPE

Poikilocytosis
Variation in shape, due to anaemia which is usually severe

Spherocytosis
Spheroidal cells seen in hereditary spherocytosis and in acquired
haemolytic anaemia

Elliptocytosis
Elliptical cells. Hereditary. Haemolytic anaemia may or may not
occur

Sickling
Crescentic cells seen when reducing agents act on Hb-S.
Hereditary.

Bizarre shapes
Seen in severe uraemia and carcinomatosis

STAINING

Hypochromia
Decreased intensity of stain, due to Fe deficiency

Polychromasia
Diffuse basophilia. Indicates active blood regeneration, just as
reticulocytosis does

Punctate basophilia
Stippled appearance seen in severe anaemia or lead poisoning

Target cells (Mexican hat cells)
Occur in:
  (i) Fe deficiency
 (ii) Liver disease
(iii) After splenectomy
(iv) Inherited Hb defect, e.g. thalassaemia major

CAUSES OF MICROCYTIC HYPOCHROMIC ANAEMIA

1. Iron deficiency
2. Thalassaemia
3. Lead poisoning
4. Some sideroblastic anaemias
5. Some anaemias of chronic disease

CAUSES OF HAEMOLYTIC ANAEMIA
CONGENITAL

1. **Spherocytosis** ('acholuric jaundice')

2. **Haemoglobinopathy:**
   (i) Sickle-cell anaemia
   (ii) Thalassaemia syndromes

3. **Metabolic defect** (enzyme defects, e.g. G6PD deficiency)

ACQUIRED

1. **Autoimmune haemolysins:**
   (i) Idiopathic warm or cold antibodies
   (ii) Viral or mycoplasmal infection

2. **Secondary (symptomatic):**
   (i) Chronic lymphocytic leukaemia
   (ii) Malignant lymphoma
   (iii) SLE
   (iv) Malaria
   (v) Uncommonly:
       Renal disease
       Liver disease
       Carcinoma
       Rheumatoid disease
       TB or syphilis

3. **Drugs and chemicals,** e.g. lead, methyldopa, dapsone

4. **Haemolytic disease of the newborn, transfusion reactions**

5. **Mechanical,** e.g. cardiac bypass surgery

6. **Microangiopathic:**
   (i) Thrombotic thrombocytopenic purpura
   (ii) Haemolytic uraemic syndrome
   (iii) Disseminated intravascular coagulation

7. **Paroxysmal nocturnal haemoglobinuria**

8. **March haemoglobinuria**

MACROCYTIC ANAEMIA
Folate comes from **Fol**iage **O**r **L**iver

CAUSES OF FOLIC ACID DEFICIENCY

1. Dietary deficiency or malabsorption
2. Pregnancy
3. Increased cell turnover, e.g. leukaemia or lymphoma
4. Anti-folate drugs, e.g. anticonvulsants, methotrexate

   B_{12} is produced by **B**acteria in animals

CAUSES OF VITAMIN B_{12} DEFICIENCY

1. Pernicious anaemia or gastrectomy
2. Changed intestinal flora, e.g. blind-loop syndrome
3. Ileal disease, e.g. Crohn's
4. Fish tape-worm (Diphyllobothrium latum) utilizes available B_{12}
5. Vegan diet

OTHER CAUSES OF MACROCYTOSIS

1. Alcoholism
2. Liver disease
3. Myxoedema
4. Post-haemorrhage (reticulocytes are large)
5. Myelodysplasia
6. Aplastic anaemia
7. Cytotoxic drugs, esp. hydroxyurea
8. Pregnancy

CLINICAL FEATURES OF ADDISONIAN PERNICIOUS ANAEMIA

1. Usually over 30, may have blue eyes, fair hair, premature greying
2. Anaemia of insidious onset
3. Glossitis, often intermittent
4. GI symptoms, e.g. dyspepsia, diarrhoea
5. Subacute combined degeneration of spinal cord
     (i) Peripheral neuropathy
    (ii) Dorso-lateral column involvement
   (iii) Mental changes ('megaloblastic madness')
    (iv) Rarely optic atrophy, nystagmus, impotence, etc.

   N.B. May be mixed upper motor neurone and lower motor neurone signs
6. Mild pyrexia
7. Slight hepatosplenomegaly
8. Retinal haemorrhage
9. Increased incidence of Ca stomach

LEUKOPENIA
CAUSES OF PANCYTOPENIA

1. Aplastic anaemia (q.v.)
2. Acute leukaemia (in subleukaemic phase) and some myelodysplasias
3. Marrow infiltration:
    (i) Malignant lymphoma
    (ii) Metastatic carcinoma
    (iii) Myelomatosis
    (iv) Myelosclerosis (in late stages)
4. Hypersplenism
5. Pernicious anaemia
6. SLE
7. Rarely, disseminated TB

CAUSES OF NEUTROPENIA SEVERE ENOUGH TO CAUSE SYMPTOMS (AGRANULOCYTOSIS)

1. Aplastic anaemia
    (i) Idiopathic
    (ii) Drugs, e.g.
        cytotoxic drugs
        phenylbutazone
        chloramphenicol
    (iii) Chemicals, e.g. benzene
    (iv) Radiation
2. Selective drug-induced neutropenia (normal Hb and platelets) e.g. thiouracil
3. Acute leukaemia (in subleukaemic phase)
4. Hypersplenism
5. Idiopathic (rare)

LEUKOCYTOSIS
CAUSES OF NEUTROPHIL LEUKOCYTOSIS

1. Bacterial infections
2. Myeloproliferative disease:
    Myeloid leukaemia
    Myelosclerosis
    Polycythaemia vera
3. Haemorrhage, especially internal
4. Tissue damage:
    Trauma (including surgery)
    Burns
    Myocardial infarction
5. Malignancy, especially necrotic tumours and hepatic metastases

6. Drugs, especially steroids
7. Collagen vascular disease, e.g. Still's juvenile chronic arthritis

CAUSES OF EOSINOPHILIA

1. Allergy
Hypersensitivity to food or drugs

2. Parasites
e.g. trichiniasis, hydatid, hookworm

3. Skin disease
  (i) Scabies
  (ii) Atopy (eczema, urticaria, hay fever, asthma)
  (iii) Dermatitis herpetiformis

4. Malignancy
Especially Hodgkin's disease

5. Hypereosinophilic syndromes (pulmonary eosinophilia)
A range of disease characterized by radiographic pulmonary
infiltrates, eosinophilia, and varying degrees of asthma and
vasculitis, e.g. Löeffler's disease and the pulmonary form of
polyarteritis nodosa

POLYCYTHAEMIA

CAUSES

Primary
Polycythaemia rubra vera

Secondary
1. Hypoxia
  (i) High altitude
  (ii) Cyanotic heart disease
  (iii) Pulmonary disease
  (iv) Obesity
2. Congenital abnormalities of haemoglobin with an abnormal
affinity for oxygen
3. Increased erythropoietin
  (i) Heavy cigarette smoking
  (ii) Kidney cyst, neoplasm or hydronephrosis
  (iii) Liver carcinoma
  (iv) Cerebellar haemangioblastoma
  (v) Massive uterine fibroma
4. Relative polycythaemia
  (i) Dehydration
  (ii) Stress

CLINICAL FEATURES OF POLYCYTHAEMIA RUBRA VERA

1. Headache, dizziness and lassitude
2. Plethoric appearance; engorged conjunctival and retinal vessels
3. Hypertension
4. Splenomegaly
5. Generalized pruritus
6. Dyspepsia due to GI vessel enlargement, or associated peptic ulcer
7. Thrombosis, e.g. cerebral, coronary or mesenteric
8. Haemorrhagic tendency
9. Peripheral ischaemia due to slow circulation or thrombosis
10. Gout

SPLENOMEGALY

CAUSES OF MASSIVE SPLENOMEGALY

1. **M**yelofibrosis
2. **I**diopathic tropical splenomegaly
3. **C**hronic myeloid leukaemia
4. **K**ala-azar
5. **S**chistosomiasis
   Mnemonic: MICKS

CAUSES OF MODERATE SPLENOMEGALY

All the causes of massive splenomegaly plus:
1. **B**lood dyscrasias, e.g. leukaemia, haemolysis, polycythaemia rubra vera
2. **L**ymphoma
3. **I**nfections, especially infectious mononucleosis, septicaemia, bacterial endocarditis and malaria
4. **P**ortal hypertension
5. **S**torage diseases, e.g. Gaucher's
   Mnemonic: BLIPS

CAUSES OF MILD SPLENOMEGALY

All the above plus:
Collagen–vascular disease
Hyperthyroidism (rarely)
Amyloidosis
Rheumatoid disease
Many systemic infections, TB, brucellosis, etc.
Sarcoidosis
Mnemonic: CHARMS

LYMPHADENOPATHY

CAUSES

1. Infections
    (i) Focal infection with regional lymphadenopathy, e.g. sepsis, TB, primary chancre
   (ii) HIV, e.g. persistent generalized lymphadenopathy
  (iii) Infectious mononucleosis
  (iv) Rubella
   (v) Secondary syphilis
  (vi) Toxoplasmosis
 (vii) Tropical infestation, e.g. filariasis

2. Lymphoma
    (i) Hodgkin's
   (ii) Non-Hodgkin's

3. Leukaemia
Usually lymphocytic (CLL or ALL)

4. Malignancy
    (i) Metastases
   (ii) Reactive changes

5. Miscellaneous
    (i) Sarcoidosis
   (ii) Langerhans cell histiocytosis (formerly called histiocytosis X)
  (iii) Chronic inflammatory skin disease
  (iv) Collagen–vascular disease, e.g. RA, SLE
   (v) Anticonvulsant drugs

CLINICAL FEATURES OF HODGKIN'S DISEASE

1. Weight loss, malaise, lassitude, night sweats
2. Fever (the periodic Pel–Ebstein pattern is uncommon)
3. Large, discrete, rubbery, asymmetrical superficial lymph nodes
4. Mediastinal or retroperitoneal node involvement
5. Hepatosplenomegaly
6. Pulmonary or pleural infiltration
7. Pain or paralysis due to pressure on nerves or spinal cord
8. Marrow infiltration with pain or pathological fracture
9. Skin:
    Pruritus
    Pigmentation
    Herpes zoster
    Nodular infiltrates
10. Infections due to decreased cell mediated immunity
11. Alcohol-induced pain

CLINICAL FEATURES OF THE 3 COMMON LEUKAEMIAS

Anaemia, constitutional symptoms (fever, malaise, weight loss) and bleeding (including purpura) occur in all 3 types but are more severe in acute leukaemia and less severe in chronic lymphocytic leukaemia

ACUTE MYELOID LEUKAEMIA

1. Occurs at any age
2. Onset may be abrupt or insidious
3. Stomatitis and pharyngitis
4. Susceptibility to infections, especially of upper respiratory tract
5. Slight lymphadenopathy (but more common in ALL)
6. Slight or moderate liver and spleen enlargement
7. Bone and joint pain, with sternal tenderness
8. Gum hypertrophy

CHRONIC MYELOID LEUKAEMIA (associated with Philadelphia chromosome)

1. Occurs in middle age
2. Insidious onset
3. Massive splenomegaly
4. Slight lymphadenopathy
5. Moderate hepatomegaly

CHRONIC LYMPHOCYTIC LEUKAEMIA

1. Occurs in late middle age, more often in males
2. Insidious onset often found accidentally
3. Moderate or marked lymphadenopathy, usually symmetrical
4. Recurrent chronic infections
5. Moderate liver and spleen enlargement
6. May be haemolytic anaemia
7. Skin lesions:
    (i) Pruritus
    (ii) Herpes zoster
    (iii) Nodular infiltrates
    (iv) Erythroderma (*l'homme rouge*)

CLINICAL FEATURES OF MULTIPLE MYELOMA

1. Progressive anaemia
2. Bone pain:
    (i) Osteolytic lesions
    (ii) Pathological fractures
    (iii) Osteomalacia (due to renal phosphate leak)

3. Bleeding, due to thrombocytopenia
4. Fever
5. Renal involvement:
   (i) acute or chronic uraemia
   (ii) Fanconi syndrome
6. Hepatomegaly, occasionally with jaundice
7. Hypercalcaemia with normal alkaline phosphatase
8. Hyperuricaemia
9. Amyloidosis
10. Neuropathy, with raised CSF protein
11. Susceptibility to infections, due to defective antibodies
12. Hyperviscosity syndrome (occasionally)

BLEEDING

May be due to defects of platelets, coagulation or vessels

PLATELETS

CAUSES OF THROMBOCYTOPENIA

1. Idiopathic thrombocytopenic purpura (autoimmune)
2. Causes of pancytopenia (p. 79)
3. Drugs, e.g. salicylates, heparin
4. Incompatible or massive blood transfusions
5. Disseminated intravascular coagulation
6. Massive haemorrhage

N.B. In thrombocytopenia, bleeding time and capillary fragility are increased, but coagulation time is *normal*

COAGULATION

Vitamin K deficiency affects coagulation factors II, VII, IX and X.

COAGULATION DISORDERS

CONGENITAL

Haemophilias
1. Haemophilia A (VIII deficiency)
2. Haemophilia B (IX deficiency, Christmas disease)
3. von Willebrand's disease

Other congenital deficiencies
Factors I, II, V, VII, X, XI, XII or XIII

ACQUIRED

1. Vitamin K deficiency
2. Liver disease

3. Anticoagulant drugs
4. Disseminated intravascular coagulation (consumption coagulopathy)
5. Massive transfusion of stored blood
6. Circulating inhibitors of coagulation

DISSEMINATED INTRAVASCULAR COAGULATION

This is characterized by excessive formulation of fibrinogen derivatives, usually due to increased proteolysis. There may be bleeding or thrombosis of any severity

CAUSES

1. 'Shock', esp. Gram-neg. septicaemia and anaphylaxis
2. Other infections, e.g. TB, viral and fungal
3. Obstetric
   Premature placental separation
   Retention of dead fetus
   Amniotic embolism
   Fetal death due to Rh incompatibility
4. Major surgery, especially with extra-corporeal shunts
5. Incompatible blood transfusion
6. Miscellaneous
   Leukaemia or carcinomatosis
   Liver, renal or prostatic disease
   Pulmonary embolism

CAUSES OF BLEEDING DUE TO SMALL VESSEL DEFECTS

CONGENITAL

1. Hereditary haemorrhagic telangiectasia (Osler–Weber–Rendu)
2. Pseudo-xanthoma elasticum
3. Ehlers–Danlos disease

ACQUIRED

1. **Infection**
   (i) Septicaemia, especially meningococcal
   (ii) Bacterial endocarditis

2. **Drugs,** e.g. corticosteroids

3. **Secondary to systemic disease** ('symptomatic')
   (i) Cushing's
   (ii) Scurvy

4. Vasculitis
(i) Henoch–Schönlein purpura
(ii) Cutaneous vasculitis
(iii) Polyarteritis nodosa

5. Miscellaneous
(i) Simple easy bruising
(ii) Senile purpura
(iii) Dermatoses, e.g. eczema
(iv) Fat embolism

SCREENING TESTS FOR A BLEEDING DISORDER

1. **Blood count and film**
   To detect leukaemia and assess platelet number, size and shape
2. **Bleeding time** (with Duke's method, normal < 7 min)
   Useful in diagnosis of von Willebrand's disease
   Also prolonged by aspirin
3. **Hess test,** with sphygmomanometer cuff at c. 100 mmHg for 5 min (N < 5 petechiae in a circle of 3 cm diameter)
4. **Prothrombin time** (N 12–15 sec)
   Tests the extrinsic system
   Prolonged by warfarin
5. **Activated partial thromboplastin time (APTT)** (N 30–45 sec)
   Tests the intrinsic system (especially VIII and IX)
   Prolonged by heparin
6. **Thrombin time** (N 10–20 sec)
   Prolonged in
   (i) Fibrinogen deficiency
   (ii) Presence of some inhibitors, e.g. heparin
7. **Assays for coagulation factor deficiency** (e.g. factor VII)
8. **Fibrin degradation products**
   Increased in fibrinolysis (e.g. disseminated intravascular coagulation)

Clinical features of bleeding disorders

Clinical feature	Coagulation disorder	Platelet disorder
Purpura	Rare	Common
Bruises	Single, deep	Multiple, superficial
Bleeding sites	Joints, muscles	Mucous membranes
Superficial cuts	Bleeding stops	Bleeding prolonged
Deep cuts	Bleeding continues despite pressure	Bleeding stops with pressure
Healing of cuts	Delayed	Normal

COMPLICATIONS OF BLOOD TRANSFUSION

1. **Febrile reactions**
   (i) Pyrogens
   (ii) Leukocyte or platelet iso-agglutinins
   (iii) Hypersensitivity to plasma
2. **Allergic reactions**
3. **Circulatory overload**
4. **Haemolysis.** Red cells of either donor or recipient may be affected
   (i) Blood group incompatibility
   (ii) Improper or overlong storage of donor blood
5. **Reaction due to infected stored blood**
6. **Disease transmission**
   (i) Viral hepatitis, HIV (AIDS virus), cytomegalovirus, Epstein–Barr virus
   (ii) Syphilis
   (iii) Malaria, toxoplasmosis
   (iv) Brucellosis
7. **Thrombophlebitis**
8. **Air embolism**
9. **Immunological sensitization by previous transfusion,** especially Rhesus sensitization
10. **Transfusion siderosis**
11. **Complications of massive transfusion**
    (i) Collapse due to cold blood
    (ii) Excess citrate (exaggerates bleeding tendency)
    (iii) Excess ammonia from stored blood (exaggerates precoma in cirrhotics)
    (iv) Excess potassium (exaggerates hyperkalaemia in uraemic patients)
    (v) Thrombocytopenia

CONDITIONS PREDISPOSING TO VENOUS THROMBOSIS

A. LOCALIZED

1. Stasis (tight bandages, senility, immobility, etc.)
2. Damaged vessel wall
   (i) Infection
   (ii) Atheroma
   (iii) Trauma (inc. fracture and pelvic surgery)

B. GENERALIZED

1. Thrombocytosis and polycythaemia
2. Prolonged bed rest
3. Pregnancy and puerperium
4. Oral contraceptives

5. Hyperviscosity of blood (dysproteinaemia or polycythaemia)
6. Low levels of antithrombin III, protein C or protein S
7. Cardiolipin antibody (lupus anticoagulant)
8. Factor V (Leiden)
9. Sickle-cell disorders
10. Malignancy
11. Nephrotic syndrome
12. Dehydration

8. Neurology

THE SENSORY SYSTEM

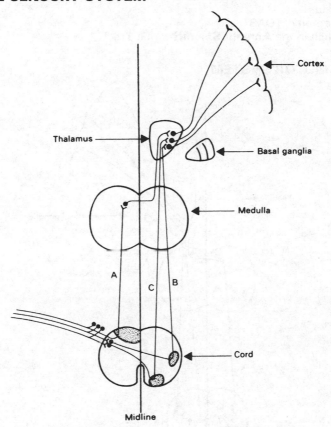

(A) Proprioception, vibration and half of touch fibres travel
via posterior nerve roots up the posterior column without relaying
in the cord. They relay in the medulla (nuclei gracilis and cuneatus)
and cross the midline to continue as the medial lemniscus to the
thalamus. Tertiary fibres travel via the posterior limb of the
internal capsule to the sensory cortex (post-central gyrus)

Mnemonic: PROVOST
PROprioception, **V**ibration and **S**oft **T**ouch in the **POST**erior column
(B) Pain and temperature fibres relay in the cord, cross the midline immediately and travel in the *lateral* spinothalamic tract to the thalamus
Mnemonic: PATEL
PAin and **TE**mp in the **L**ateral spinothalamic tract
(C) Remainder of touch fibres relay and cross the midline in the cord and travel in the *anterior* spinothalamic tract to the thalamus
Mnemonic: TOAST
TOuch in the **A**nterior **S**pinothalamic **T**ract

THE MOTOR SYSTEM

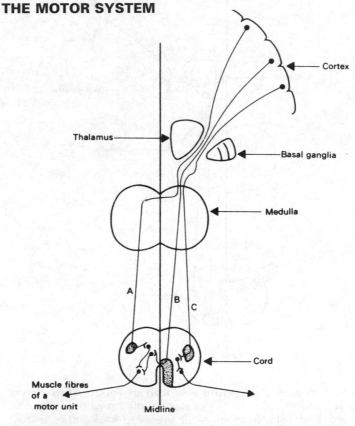

Fibres pass downwards from the motor cortex (pre-central gyrus) into the posterior limb of the internal capsule. In the pons the fibres are scattered, but they regroup on the upper medulla to form protuberances called the pyramids

(A) In the lower medulla the majority of fibres decussate and descend in the *lateral* corticospinal (crossed pyramidal) tracts

(B) Some fibres do not decussate, but descend in the *anterior* corticospinal tract, and then cross in the anterior commissure of the cord to supply muscles in the neck

(C) A few fibres descend directly in the *lateral* corticospinal tract with the crossed fibres from the contralateral cortex

Most fibres relay with internuncial cells in the cord, and the anterior horn cells and their fibres then form the 'final common pathway' to the motor end-plates in the muscle. The organization of movement is much more complex than this diagram suggests, since impulses are modified by the cerebellum, the extrapyramidal system and proprioceptive and other sensations

Mnemonic: MOLAC

MOtor in **L**ateral, **A**nterior and **C**ontralateral tracts

SIGNS OF A LOWER MOTOR NEURONE LESION

1. Weakness and wasting
2. Hypotonicity
3. Decreased reflexes
4. Fasciculation

SIGNS OF AN UPPER MOTOR NEURONE LESION

1. Weakness
2. Spasticity
3. Increased tendon reflexes, sometimes with clonus
4. Extensor plantar response

N.B. In pyramidal (UMN) lesions, the extensors are weaker than the flexors in the arms, but the reverse is true in the legs, thus accounting for the 'spastic' posture

CRANIAL NERVE SUPPLY

1. **Olfactory.** Smell
2. **Optic.** Vision
3. **Oculomotor**
   (i) All ocular muscles, except superior oblique and lateral rectus
   (ii) Ciliary muscle
   (iii) Sphincter pupillae
   (iv) Levator palpebrae superioris
4. **Trochlear.** Superior oblique muscle
   N.B. Tested by asking patient to look down and *inwards*
5. **Trigeminal**
   (i) Sensory for face, cornea, sinuses, nasal mucosa, teeth, tympanic membrane and anterior two-thirds of tongue
   (ii) Motor to muscles of mastication

6. **Abducens.**   Lateral rectus muscle
7. **Facial**
     (i) Motor to scalp and facial muscles of expression
     (ii) Taste in anterior two-thirds of tongue (via chorda
          tympani)
     (iii) Nerve to stapedius muscle
8. **Auditory.**   Auditory and vestibular components
9. **Glossopharyngeal**
     (i) Sensory for posterior one-third of tongue, pharynx and
          middle ear
     (ii) Taste fibres for posterior one-third of tongue
     (iii) Motor to middle constrictor of pharynx and
          stylopharyngeus
10. **Vagal**
     (i) Motor to soft palate, larynx and pharynx (from nucleus
          ambiguus)
     (ii) Sensory and motor for heart, respiratory passages and
          abdominal viscera (from dorsal nucleus)
11. **Spinal accessory**
     (i) Motor to sternomastoid and trapezius
     (ii) Accessory fibres to vagus
12. **Hypoglossal.**   Motor to tongue and hyoid bone depressors

CRANIAL NERVE NUCLEI

Mid-brain   3, 4
Pons   5, 6, 7, 8
Medulla   9, 10, 11, 12

OPTIC PATHWAY AND PATTERNS OF VISUAL FIELD LOSS

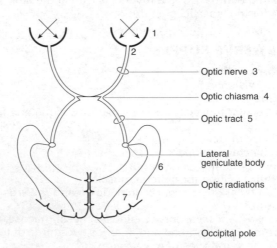

Optic nerve 3

Optic chiasma 4

Optic tract 5

Lateral geniculate body

Optic radiations

Occipital pole

1. Concentric diminution ('tunnel vision')

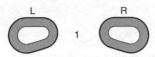

Chronic glaucoma, retinitis pigmentosa
Chronic papilloedema can occasionally cause irregular loss of
peripheral visual fields
In acute papilloedema there is usually no field defect, though
the blind spot may be enlarged.

2. Central scotoma

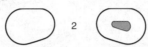

Retinal disease involving macula, retrobulbar neuritis

3. Complete field loss in one eye

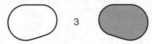

Optic nerve lesion (i.e. anterior to chiasma)

4. Bitemporal hemianopia

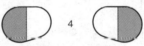

Pituitary tumour (i.e. at the chiasma)

5. Homonymous hemianopia

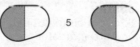

Tract lesions posterior to chiasma

6. Quadrantic hemianopia

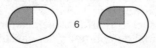

Temporal lobe tumours for superior quadrant
Parietal lobe tumours for inferior quadrant

7. Homonymous hemianopia with macular sparing

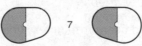

Lesions of the visual cortex

CAUSES OF OPTIC ATROPHY

1. **Glaucoma**
2. **Retinal lesions**
   Choroido-retinitis
   Intra-ocular haemorrhage, etc.
3. **Optic neuritis** (retrobulbar neuritis) (q.v.)
4. **Chronic papilloedema**
5. **Pressure on optic nerve**
   Tumour
   Aneurysm
   Paget's disease
6. **Division of optic nerve**
   Surgery
   Trauma

CAUSES OF OPTIC NEURITIS

1. **Ischaemia**
   e.g. temporal arteritis
2. **Demyelinating disease**
   e.g. multiple sclerosis
3. **Infective**
   e.g. retinitis, meningitis
4. **Toxins**
   e.g. methyl alcohol
5. **Metabolic**
   e.g. diabetes mellitus, B_{12} deficiency

FEATURES OF DIABETIC RETINOPATHY

1. **Background retinopathy**
   Microaneurysms leak, producing 'dot and blot' haemorrhages
   and, some years later, hard exudates
2. **Pre-proliferative retinopathy**
   Soft exudates (cotton-wool spots) appear. These are deep
   retinal infarcts. Venous dilatation and bleeding occurs
3. **Proliferative retinopathy**
   Extensive new vessel formation which can lead to vitreous
   haemorrhage, retinal detachment, neovascular glaucoma, etc.

FEATURES OF HYPERTENSIVE RETINOPATHY

Grade 1. Silver-wiring of arteries
Grade 2. Arteriovenous nipping
Grade 3. Flame-shaped haemorrhages, exudates and cotton-wool
spots
Grade 4. As Grade 3, but with papilloedema

SQUINTS

CONCOMITANT SQUINT

Due to a defect in the sensory component of the reflex arc (such as poor vision) or a central disturbance. The angle of deviation between the eyes remains constant when looking in different directions. This occurs in all neonates and often in childhood following illness

Features
1. Both eyes have full movement if tested separately
2. No diplopia

PARALYTIC SQUINT

Due to lesions of 3rd, 4th or 6th cranial nerves. Usually causes diplopia

Features
1. 'False' image is always peripheral
2. 'False' image is seen by affected eye
3. Separation of images is maximal when looking in direction of action of affected muscle

3RD CRANIAL NERVE (OCULOMOTOR) PALSY

1. Marked ptosis
2. Eye abducted and depressed ('down and out')
3. Pupil **dilated** and completely non-reactive

   More often partial than complete, especially with lesions near the nucleus

Causes of oculomotor palsy
1. Aneurysm of posterior communicating artery
2. Tumours
3. Brain-stem CVA

CERVICAL SYMPATHETIC PARALYSIS (HORNER'S)

1. Mild ptosis
2. Pupil **constricted** with no reaction to shading
3. Reduced sweating on ipsilateral half of head and neck
4. Abolition of ciliospinal reflex

   N.B. Everything gets 'smaller'

Causes of Horner's syndrome
1. Carcinoma of apical bronchus (Pancoast's tumour)
2. Cervical sympathectomy
3. Aortic aneurysm

4. Syringobulbia or syringomyelia
5. Brachial plexus lesions (e.g. Klumpke's paralysis)

CAUSES OF PTOSIS

1. Congenital
2. Oculomotor palsy
3. Cervical sympathetic lesion
4. Myasthenia gravis
5. Myopathy (e.g. dystrophia myotonica)

PAPILLOEDEMA

SIGNS OF PAPILLOEDEMA

1. Engorged retinal veins
2. Pink disc with blurred margin
3. Loss of 'cupping'
4. Cribrosa not visible
5. Flame-shaped haemorrhages

COMMON CAUSES OF PAPILLOEDEMA

1. Accelerated phase hypertension
2. Raised intracranial pressure (q.v.)
3. Retinal venous obstruction

Papillitis (retrobulbar neuritis) is usually due to disseminated sclerosis. It is distinguished by the early severe loss of visual acuity. There may be no fundal abnormality (i.e. 'patient sees nothing, doctor sees nothing')

Causes of raised intracranial pressure
1. Intracranial mass or infection
2. Obstructed CSF flow
3. Hypertensive encephalopathy
4. Hypercapnia (CO_2 retention)
5. Benign intracranial hypertension (pseudo-tumour cerebri)
    (i) Thrombosis of intracranial venous sinuses
    (ii) Many rare causes, e.g. oral contraceptives, retinoids or vitamin A poisoning

CAUSES OF SUDDEN BLINDNESS

1. Retinal detachment
2. Acute glaucoma
3. Vitreous haemorrhage (esp. diabetes)
4. Temporal arteritis
5. Retinal artery or vein occlusion
6. Migraine (transient)

CAUSES OF FACIAL PARALYSIS

1. SUPRANUCLEAR LESIONS

   e.g. cerebrovascular accident affecting internal capsule

2. NUCLEAR LESIONS

   e.g. pontine neoplasm, polio

3. INFRANUCLEAR LESIONS

   (i) Cerebello-pontine angle and internal auditory canal, e.g. acoustic neuroma, meningioma
   (ii) Facial canal, e.g. Bell's palsy, trauma, sarcoidosis
   (iii) Extra-cranial, e.g. trauma, parotid neoplasm

   In upper motor neurone facial palsy the forehead movements are retained (due to bilateral cortical representation)

DEAFNESS

CAUSES OF DEAFNESS

A. Conduction deafness
1. Wax or foreign body
2. Eustachian obstruction (esp. 'glue ear')
3. Otitis media
4. Otosclerosis
5. Paget's disease

B. Nerve deafness
1. Traumatic:
   (i) Chronic exposure to loud noise
   (ii) Fracture of petrous temporal bone
2. Infective:
   (i) Congenital syphilis
   (ii) Rubella syndrome
   (iii) Mumps, influenza
3. Toxic:
   (i) Aspirin, quinine
   (ii) Antibiotics e.g. streptomycin, neomycin
   (iii) Tobacco, alcohol
4. Degenerative:
   Presbyacusis
5. Tumour, e.g. acoustic neuroma
6. Brain-stem lesions (rarely)
7. Rare familial syndromes

RINNE'S TEST

The ability to hear a tuning fork through air and through the mastoid process are compared. In *normal* people and in *nerve* deafness the air conducted sound is louder, whereas in conduction deafness it is softer

WEBER'S TEST

The base of the fork is placed on the centre of the forehead; in *nerve* deafness the note is heard in the *normal* ear, whereas in conduction deafness it is heard in the deaf ear

MULTIPLE SCLEROSIS

Characterized by multiple CNS lesions scattered in time and place
   Lower motor neurones are not affected directly

CLINICAL FEATURES

1. Spastic weakness, usually starting in legs
2. Retrobulbar neuritis:
   Misty vision
   Painful eye movements
   Slightly swollen optic disc
   Central scotoma
   (Optic atrophy may develop)
3. Numbness and paraesthesiae
4. Diplopia (ataxic nystagmus is characteristic)
5. Vertigo
6. Cerebellar signs:
   'Scanning' speech
   Intention tremor
   Nystagmus (may be worse in the abducting eye)
7. Sphincter disturbance and impotence
8. Euphoria or other mental change
9. Painful flexor spasms

INTRACRANIAL DISORDERS

COMMON INTRACRANIAL NEOPLASMS

Children
Medulloblastoma
Astrocytoma

Adults
Metastatic cancer
Glioma
Meningioma

Acoustic neuroma
Pituitary tumour

CLINICAL FEATURES OF INTRACRANIAL NEOPLASM

1. Raised intracranial pressure
   (i) Headache, worse on straining and on waking
   (ii) Drowsiness
   (iii) Bradycardia and hypertension
   (iv) Vomiting
   (v) Papilloedema
2. Progressive loss of neurological function or focal neurological signs (q.v.)
3. Epilepsy
4. Mental symptoms, e.g. personality change, apathy, dementia
5. Coning may occur, with dilated pupil and respiratory depression (may follow bleed into tumour)

LOCALIZATION OF CORTICAL LESIONS BY FOCAL NEUROLOGICAL SIGNS

Frontal
1. Mental disturbance
   (i) Dementia
   (ii) Apathy
   (iii) Inappropriate emotion
2. Epilepsy
3. Grasp reflex
4. Unilateral anosmia

Pre-central
1. Jacksonian epilepsy
2. Contralateral spastic hemiplegia

Parietal
1. Sensory disturbance, e.g. lack of 2 point discrimination
2. Visual aphasia
3. Homonymous hemianopia or quadrantanopia (lower)
4. Apraxia
5. Astereognosis

Temporal
1. Anterior lesions — motor aphasia
   Posterior lesions — auditory aphasia
2. Homonymous hemianopia or quadrantanopia (upper)
3. Psychomotor epilepsy

Occipital
Visual field defects

SIGNS OF A CEREBELLAR LESION

1. Intention tremor
2. 'Scanning' speech
3. Nystagmus worse on looking to the side of the lesion
4. Limb ataxia with characteristic broad-based gait
5. Hypotonia and pendular reflexes

CAUSES OF CEREBELLAR DYSFUNCTION

1. Multiple sclerosis
2. Neoplasms
    (i) In the cerebellum, e.g. medulloblastoma
    (ii) Paraneoplastic neuropathy, e.g. due to bronchial cancer
3. Cerebellar abscess (often secondary to otitis media)
4. Vertebrobasilar insufficiency
5. Drugs, e.g. alcohol
6. Idiopathic degeneration, e.g. primary cerebellar atrophy
7. Rare hereditary and familial ataxias, e.g. Friedreich's

CLASSIFICATION OF SPEECH DEFECTS

1. Dysphasia (disorder in use of symbols for communication whether spoken, heard, written or read)
2. Dysarthria (disorder of articulation)
3. Dysphonia (disorder of vocalization)
4. Dementia (intellectual deterioration)

CAUSES OF DYSPHASIA

1. Expressive — due to lesion of **B**roca's area (**I**nferior **F**rontal gyrus of dominant cortex)
   Mnemonic: BIF and BROca BROadcasts
2. Receptive — due to lesion of **WE**rnicke's area (**S**uperior **T**emporal areas of dominant cortex)
   Mnemonic: WEST

CAUSES OF DYSARTHRIA

1. Bulbar or pseudo-bulbar palsy
2. Basal ganglia lesions
3. Cerebellar lesions
4. Weakness or paralysis of facial muscles
5. Oral lesions including loose dentures

CAUSES OF DYSPHONIA

1. Functional (hysteria)

2. Lesions of recurrent laryngeal nerve (Ca bronchus, aortic aneurysm)
3. Vocal cord lesion (infection, tumour, etc.)

CAUSES OF CEREBRAL INFARCTION

1. Atheroma of intra- or extracranial arteries
2. Cerebral emboli:
   (i) Atrial fibrillation
   (ii) Myocardial infarct
   (iii) Bacterial endocarditis
   (iv) Fat embolism
3. Cerebral ischaemia due to severe hypotension
4. Cerebral arterial spasm, e.g. migraine or following subarachnoid haemorrhage
5. Hypoxia, e.g.
   (i) Cardiac arrest
   (ii) Carbon monoxide poisoning
   (iii) Pulmonary emboli
6. Arteritis, e.g. collagen–vascular disease
7. Cerebral thrombosis, e.g. due to polycythaemia
8. Dissecting aortic aneurysm involving the carotid artery
9. Ligation of carotid artery for intracranial aneurysm

SUBARACHNOID HAEMORRHAGE

(Sub**AR**achnoid is **AR**terial)

COMMON CAUSES

1. Ruptured 'berry' aneurysm (70%)
2. Arteriovenous malformation (10%)

CLINICAL FEATURES

1. Often occurs in middle life
2. Sudden onset of catastrophic headache, usually occipital. Often precipitated by straining. Often 'warning' headaches in previous weeks
3. Small leakages — delirium or confusion but no loss of consciousness
   Bigger bleeds — vomiting, convulsions and coma
4. Meningism
5. Plantar responses are usually extensor
6. May be slow pulse, or hypertension
7. Occasionally squint, papilloedema, retinal haemorrhage and small sluggish pupils. The characteristic subhyaloid haemorrhage spreads out from the edge of the disc
8. May be pain in back due to blood in spinal theca
9. May be pyrexia

CHRONIC SUBDURAL HAEMATOMA

CAUSE

Rupture of cortical veins as they cross the subdural space. May be traumatic or spontaneous

CLINICAL FEATURES

1. Often elderly patients, after a trivial head injury. Also in infants or alcoholics
2. Latent period of days or months occurs before symptoms develop
3. Gradual onset of headaches, memory loss, dementia, confusion, drowsiness and eventual coma. Symptoms fluctuate from day to day, with lucid intervals
4. May be signs of an intracranial space-occupying lesion, with localizing signs

EXTRADURAL HAEMATOMA

(Ex**TRA**dural is **ART**erial)

CAUSE

Fracture of squamous temporal bone with rupture of a branch of the middle meningeal artery

CLINICAL FEATURES

1. Any age, but often young adults with scalp oedema above the ear
2. Concussion may be followed by recovery of consciousness for minutes or hours before the onset of drowsiness and deepening coma
3. Signs of intracranial compression (p. 99)
4. Ipsilateral 3rd nerve palsy due to cerebral herniation
5. Progressive contralateral hemiplegia
   The signs develop rapidly and immediate operation to relieve the pressure is mandatory

CAUSES OF COMA

1. Syncope (q.v.)
2. Head injury
3. Epilepsy
4. Drugs or toxins (especially alcohol or 'overdose')
5. CVA (thrombosis, embolism or haemorrhage)
6. Raised intracranial pressure (p. 96)
7. Metabolic

    (i) Hypoglycaemia
   (ii) Diabetic ketoacidaemia
  (iii) Hepatic, renal or adrenal failure
  (iv) Myxoedema
   (v) Electrolyte imbalance
8. Acute CNS infection, e.g. meningitis, encephalitis
9. Acute systemic infection, e.g. septicaemia
10. Hysteria, hypnosis
11. Hypo- or hyperthermia

SYNCOPE ('BLACK-OUT')

A transient loss of consciousness caused by cerebral anoxia,
usually due to inadequate blood flow

CAUSES

1. Vasovagal
    (i) Emotion, heat or standing still
   (ii) Loss of blood or plasma
  (iii) Postural hypotension, e.g. drugs or prolonged
       recumbency
  (iv) Carotid sinus hypersensitivity

2. Cardiac
    (i) Stokes–Adams (heart block)
   (ii) Ventricular tachycardia or fibrillation
  (iii) Aortic stenosis
  (iv) Cyanotic congenital heart disease (fall in Po_2)
   (v) Cough syncope (obstructed venous return to heart)

3. Arterial occlusion
    (i) Atheroma or embolism (carotid or vertebrobasilar)
   (ii) Cervical spondylosis
  (iii) Strangulation
  (iv) 'Subclavian steal syndrome'

4. Anoxaemia
    (i) High altitude
   (ii) Anaemia

EPILEPSY

Partial seizures (with a single cortical focus) may be either:
Simple (unimpaired consciousness) or
Complex (impaired consciousness)

Partial seizures may progress to become **generalized**

CAUSES OF EPILEPSY

1. IDIOPATHIC
2. FOCAL CEREBRAL LESIONS
    (i) Birth injury or cerebral malformation
    (ii) Tumour
    (iii) Trauma, scar, irradiation, atrophy
    (iv) Vascular
        CVA
        Hypertension
        Vasculitis, e.g. SLE
        Vascular malformation (e.g. Sturge–Weber)
    (v) Infection
        Encephalitis or meningitis
        Abscess or tuberculoma
        Syphilis (GPI or gumma)
        Hydatid cysts, cysticercosis or toxoplasmosis
    (iv) Degenerative disease, e.g. presenile dementia

3. METABOLIC
    (i) Pyrexia in children
    (ii) Anoxia, hypoglycaemia or hypocalcaemia
    (iii) Electrolyte imbalance, e.g. water intoxication
    (iv) Uraemia
    (v) Hepatic coma
    (vi) Drugs and toxins
        Lead poisoning
        Withdrawal of alcohol or barbiturates
        'Overdose' (e.g. antidepressants)

CAUSES OF DEMENTIA

PRIMARY PRESENILE OR SENILE DEMENTIA

Idiopathic cerebral atrophy, Alzheimer's, Huntington's, etc.

SECONDARY

A. Intra-cranial
1. Tumour, especially frontal
2. Subdural haematoma
3. Vascular, especially atheroma or multiple small emboli
4. Infections, e.g. AIDS, encephalitis, neurosyphilis, Creutzfeldt–Jakob
5. Trauma (including concussion in boxers)
6. Multiple sclerosis
7. Normal pressure hydrocephalus

B. Extra-cranial
1. Metabolic (anoxia, hypoglycaemia, liver failure, renal failure)
2. Hypothyroidism
3. Vitamin deficiency (especially B_{12})
4. Drugs (especially barbiturates)
5. Toxins, especially alcohol, lead and aluminium

Depression may cause pseudodementia

NEUROLOGICAL MANIFESTATIONS OF AIDS

1. FUNCTIONAL

   Anxiety, depression, etc., which may lead to suicide

2. FOCAL INFECTION OR MENINGITIS

   Especially with opportunistic organisms:
   (i) Cryptococcus (meningitis)
   (ii) Toxoplasmosis (abscess or encephalitis)
   (iii) Cytomegalovirus (encephalitis)
   (iv) Progressive multifocal leucoencephalopathy (now thought to be due to a virus)

3. PRIMARY HIV INFECTION

   (i) Acute encephalopathy at time of seroconversion:
        May be EEG changes and epilepsy
   (ii) AIDS-dementia complex with paraparesis and incontinence
   (iii) Myelopathy due to HIV

4. OTHER

   Cerebral lymphoma, cranial or peripheral neuropathy, or myopathy

CAUSES OF PARKINSONISM

1. Idiopathic (especially over 50)
2. Cerebral atheroma
3. Drugs (e.g. phenothiazines)
4. Toxins, e.g. manganese, copper, carbon monoxide, kernicterus
5. Trauma (e.g. boxing)
6. Post-encephalitic (encephalitis lethargica outbreaks occurred 1917–1925)
7. Rare syndromes: Shy–Drager, Wilson's, Steele–Richardson

CLINICAL FEATURES OF PARKINSONISM

Characteristic tremor, rigidity and bradykinesia

1. Slowness and poverty of spontaneous movement
2. Coarse tremor ('pill-rolling') with cogwheel rigidity
3. Expressionless, unblinking face
4. Shuffling gait (festination later) with lack of arm-swinging
5. Slurred, monotonous speech and small handwriting
6. Increased salivation and dribbling
7. Oculogyric crises (forced upward deviation of eyes) in drug-induced and post-encephalitic types

ABNORMAL GAITS

N.B. Most cases are due to lesions of bone, joint or skin

'NEUROLOGICAL' GAITS

1. **Upper motor neurone hemiplegia**
   Arm adducted and internally rotated
   Elbow flexed and pronated
   Fingers flexed
   Foot plantar-flexed, with leg swung in a lateral arc

2. **Spastic paraplegia**
   Stiff jerky 'scissors' gait, with complicated assisting movements of upper limbs

3. **Parkinsonism**
   Small shuffling hurried steps
   Flexion of neck, elbows, wrists and MP joints with thumbs adducted

4. **Cerebellar lesion**
   'Drunken' gait on a broad base. Feet raised excessively and placed carefully, with patient looking ahead. Tends to fall to side of lesion

5. **Posterior column lesion**
   Patient walks on a broad base but bangs feet down clumsily and tends to look at feet. Rombergism is present

6. **High stepping gait**
   Due to foot drop

7. **Proximal myopathy**
   Waddling gait with broad base, lordosis and marked body swing. This gait occurs also in congenital hip dislocation and pregnancy

8. **Hysterical**
   Usually bizarre and inconsistent, and the patient rarely falls

9. **Involuntary movements**
     (i) *Choreiform* — jerky movements of short duration, affecting limbs and face
    (ii) *Athetoid* — slow writhing of arms and legs with flexed fingers, thumb and wrist
   (iii) *Dystonia musculorum* (torsion spasm) — intense sustained spasm of proximal and trunk muscles may cause bizarre stepping or bowing of the trunk
    (iv) *Hemiballismus* — unilateral forceful throwing movements which are almost continuous

SYRINGOMYELIA AND SYRINGOBULBIA

SYRINGOMYELIA

Usually starts in base of posterior horn or cervical region

Clinical features
Insidious onset of
1. Weakness and wasting of small muscles of hand
2. Dissociated sensory loss in hand (pain and temperature only)
3. Trophic changes:
     (i) Cyanosis of fingers
    (ii) Ulceration and scarring
   (iii) Swollen fingers due to subcutaneous hypertrophy
4. Loss of tendon reflexes
5. Painful arm
6. Spastic paraplegia
7. Charcot joints (neck and shoulders)

SYRINGOBULBIA

Medulla may be initial site, or may be involved by upward extension from cord

Clinical features
1. Facial pain or sensory loss (Cr. 5)
2. Vertigo and nystagmus (Cr. 8)
3. Facial, palatal or laryngeal palsy (Cr. 7, 9, 10, 11)
4. Wasted tongue (Cr. 12)
5. Horner's syndrome (sympathetic)

BULBAR PALSY

Bilateral *lower* motor neurone lesions of the bulbar nuclei (9, 10, 11 and 12 with lowermost part of 7)
   Mnemonic: **B**u**L**bar = **B**ilat. **L**ower

CLINICAL FEATURES

1. Dysarthria
2. Dysphagia, especially with fluids
3. Wasted fibrillating tongue
4. Palatal paralysis

CAUSES

1. Motor neurone disease
2. Polio
3. Encephalitis
4. Syringobulbia

PSEUDO-BULBAR PALSY

Bilateral *upper* motor neurone lesions of the same nuclei
   Mnemonic: P**S**eudo-bulbar is **S**uperior

CLINICAL FEATURES

1. Dysarthria
2. Dysphagia
3. Spastic tongue
4. Exaggerated jaw-jerk (spastic masseters)
5. Emotional liability

CAUSES

1. Ischaemia of internal capsule
2. Motor neurone disease
3. Disseminated sclerosis

SPINAL CORD COMPRESSION

SYMPTOMS

1. Root pains occur early. Often precipitated by movement or straining
2. Progressive weakness, paraesthesiae and sensory loss
3. Sphincter disturbances occur at a late stage

SIGNS

1. Lower motor neurone signs at level of compression and spasticity below
2. Sensory or reflex 'level'. May be hyperaesthesia at the affected level
3. Loss of abdominal reflexes in thoracic or cervical lesions

CAUSES OF CORD COMPRESSION

1. **Vertebral**
   - (i) Metastatic cancer (esp. bronchus, breast, prostate)
   - (ii) Osteoporotic collapse
   - (iii) Pott's disease (TB)
   - (iv) Spondylosis with disc prolapse
   - (v) Trauma (fracture, dislocation)

2. **Extra-dural**
   - (i) Abscess

3. **Intra-dural**
   - (i) Infiltration of meninges — lymphoma, leukaemia
   - (ii) Extra-medullary tumours — meningioma, neurofibroma
   - (iii) Intra-medullary tumours — glioma
   - (iv) Inflammation — transverse myelitis

CAUSES OF ROOT LESIONS

1. Disc protrusion
2. Spondylosis (osteophyte)
3. Metastatic cancer

CLINICAL FEATURES OF ROOT LESIONS

1. Pain in the appropriate myotome, aggravated by straining
2. Paraesthesiae in the dermatome
3. Spinal muscle spasm, e.g. lumbar scoliosis or restriction of neck movement
4. Weakness, wasting and fasciculation of the myotome, with decreased tendon reflex

DERMATOMES AND MYOTOMES

DERMATOMES OF HEAD AND NECK

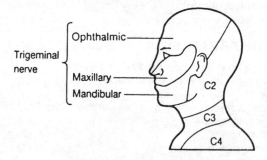

Dermatomes in the lower limb

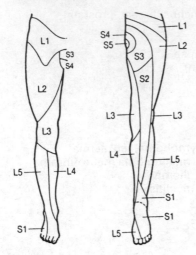

Dermatomes in the upper limb

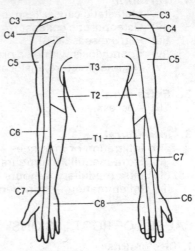

MYOTOMES WORTH REMEMBERING

C6 — Biceps, brachioradialis, radial extensors of wrist
C7 — Triceps, ulnar extensors of wrist, finger extensors
C8 — Finger flexors
L4 — Quadriceps femoris
L5 — Extensor hallucis longus
S1 — Plantar flexors

REFLEXES

Ankle jerk   S1, 2
Knee   L3, 4
Biceps   C5, 6
Triceps   C7, 8
   (Start low and work up)

CAUSES OF PARAPLEGIA

1. Hereditary spastic paraplegia
2. Cerebral birth injury (cerebral palsy)
3. Trauma
4. Cord compression — intra- or extramedullary (p. 109)
5. Multiple sclerosis
6. Syringomyelia
7. Motor neurone disease

8. Poliomyelitis
9. Sub-acute combined degeneration
10. Guillain–Barré (acute post-infective polyneuritis)

PERIPHERAL NEUROPATHY

Characterized by symmetrical flaccid weakness and sensory changes of 'glove and stocking' distribution

CAUSES OF POLYNEUROPATHY

1. **Many cases are idiopathic**

2. **Drugs and chemicals**
   Vincristine, amiodarone, mercury
   Lead causes motor neuropathy
   Isoniazid (via pyridoxine deficiency)
   Many organic chemicals

3. *Metabolic*
   Diabetes mellitus
   Amyloidosis
   Acute intermittent porphyria
   Uraemia
   Myxoedema

4. **Deficiency states**
   B_{12} deficiency
   Alcoholism
   Beri-beri (thiamine deficiency)
   Pellagra (nicotinamide deficiency)

5. **Infections**
   Leprosy
   Diphtheria
   Tetanus
   Botulism

6. **Miscellaneous**
   'Acute infective polyneuritis' of Guillain–Barré
   Collagen–vascular disease, esp. polyarteritis and rheumatoid disease
   Malignancy
   Sarcoidosis

7. **Congenital**
   Rare hereditary ataxias and neuropathies (e.g. Charcot–Marie–Tooth)

CAUSES OF PROXIMAL MYOPATHY

CONGENITAL

Muscular dystrophy

RHEUMATIC

Polymyalgia rheumatica
Polymyositis or dermatomyositis

METABOLIC

Diabetes mellitus
Glucocorticoids (Cushing's or iatrogenic)
Osteomalacia
Thyrotoxicosis or myxoedema
Carcinomatous neuromyopathy

9. Endocrinology

THE PITUITARY
PITUITARY HORMONES
Anterior
FSH, LH, ACTH, TSH, Growth hormone, Prolactin
Mnemonic: FLAT GP

Posterior
ADH
Oxytocin

PITUITARY SPACE-OCCUPYING LESIONS
1. Secreting adenomas
    (i) Prolactinoma
    (ii) Cushing's (ACTH)
    (iii) Acromegaly (GH)
2. Non-secreting adenomas
3. Craniopharyngioma
4. Metastatic carcinoma or lymphoma
5. Granuloma, e.g. sarcoid, TB

PRESENTATION OF PITUITARY LESIONS
1. Symptoms due to excess secretion of hormones
    (i) Prolactin — amenorrhoea, galactorrhoea, hirsutism
    (ii) ACTH — Cushing's disease
    (iii) GH — acromegaly
2. Hypopituitarism due to destruction of normal pituitary tissue
3. Headache
4. Visual field defects, usually bitemporal hemianopia
5. Pituitary apoplexy (rare)

CLINICAL FEATURES OF ACROMEGALY
Symptoms
1. Often insidious, with no symptoms
2. Headaches
3. Paraesthesiae (median nerve compression)
4. Proximal weakness and joint pains

5. Polyuria
6. Impotence and loss of libido in men
7. Hirsutism and amenorrhoea in women
8. Visual deterioration
9. Galactorrhoea

Signs
 1. Characteristic facies, large hands, feet and tongue
 2. Leathery furrowed skin. May be seborrhoea, hyperhidrosis or pigmentation
 3. Hoarse deep voice
 4. Non-toxic goitre
 5. Gynaecomastia
 6. Bitemporal hemianopia, optic atrophy, ocular palsies
 7. Generalized organomegaly
 8. Cardiac failure (hypertension and ischaemia)
 9. Signs of diabetes mellitus or its complications
10. Hypopituitarism
11. Progressive kyphosis
12. Arthropathy

HYPOPITUITARISM

CAUSES

1. Tumours:
    (i) Chromophobe adenoma
    (ii) Eosinophil adenoma (basophil adenoma is rarely large enough to cause hypopituitarism)
    (iii) Craniopharyngioma
    (iv) Metastatic cancer
2. Iatrogenic — hypophysectomy or irradiation
3. Pituitary necrosis due to ante- or postpartum haemorrhage (Sheehan's syndrome)
4. Granulomatous infiltration, e.g. sarcoidosis
5. Trauma
6. Infection, e.g. TB, meningitis

CLINICAL FEATURES

Loss of anterior pituitary hormones is usually partial, in the following order of frequency:

1. Somatotrophin (GH):
    (i) Dwarfism in children
    (ii) Insulin sensitivity in adults

2. Prolactin:
    Failure of lactation in postpartum patients

3. **Gonadotrophins (LH and FSH):**
   (i) Delayed puberty in children
   (ii) Loss of body hair, fine wrinkled skin, impotence, infertility and amenorrhoea in adults

4. **Thyrotrophin (TSH):**
   Hypothyroidism

5. **Corticotrophin (ACTH):**
   Hypoadrenalism (asthenia, nausea, vomiting, hypoglycaemia, collapse)

6. **Melanocyte-stimulating hormone (MSH):**
   Skin pallor

THE THYROID
HYPOTHYROIDISM
CAUSES
Primary (thyroid gland failure)
1. Autoimmune thyroiditis (Hashimoto's disease and its atrophic variant, myxoedema). In Hashimoto's the thyroid is large and may be tender, but in myxoedema it is impalpable. Circulating thyroid antibodies occur in both
2. Iatrogenic:
   (i) Surgery
   (ii) Irradiation
   (iii) Antithyroid drugs
   (iv) Lithium
3. Endemic cretinism (maternal iodine deficiency)
4. Absence or maldevelopment of thyroid gland (rare)
5. Dyshormonogenesis (rare congenital enzyme defects affecting hormone synthesis)

Secondary (TSH deficiency)
1. Pituitary lesion
2. Rarely hypothalamic lesion (due to thyrotrophin releasing hormone deficiency)

CLINICAL FEATURES
1. Mental and physical sluggishness
2. Cold intolerance
3. Constipation
4. Weight gain
5. Croaking voice, with slow speech
6. Rough, dry yellowish skin

7. 'Myxoedema facies' with generalized thickening of subcutaneous tissue, periorbital puffiness, brittle sparse hair and thin eyebrows
8. Bradycardia
9. Delayed relaxation of tendon jerks

Less commonly
10. Anaemia (may be macrocytic)
11. Cyanosis, Raynaud's phenomenon or angina
12. Carpal tunnel syndrome
13. Perceptive deafness
14. Myalgia or arthralgia
15. 'Myxoedema madness'
16. Coma

ORGAN-SPECIFIC AUTOIMMUNE DISEASES

1. Hashimoto's thyroiditis
2. Adrenalitis (Addison's)
3. Pernicious anaemia
4. Juvenile-onset diabetes mellitus
5. Vitiligo
6. ?Alopecia areata

CAUSES OF 'NON-TOXIC' GOITRE

1. 'Simple' colloid goitre (idiopathic), common during puberty and pregnancy
2. Diffuse multinodular goitre (may become toxic)
3. Iodine deficiency
4. Goitrogens, e.g. antithyroid drugs, excess iodine
5. Autoimmune thyroiditis (Hashimoto's)

Possibility of malignancy is suggested by:
1. Asymmetrical enlargement with 'cold area' on scan
2. Very hard thyroid
3. Pressure effects, e.g. hoarseness
4. Cervical lymphadenopathy

HYPERTHYROIDISM

CAUSES

1. Graves' disease
2. Toxic multinodular goitre. Resembles Graves' disease but patients tend to be older, with fewer eye signs
3. Toxic adenoma
4. Iatrogenic (excess thyroid hormone)

CLINICAL FEATURES OF GRAVES' DISEASE

Thyroid gland
1. Goitre, usually diffuse (but may be nodular)
2. Increased thyroid vascularity (thrill, bruit)

Metabolic
3. Increased heat production (warm moist skin, heat intolerance)
4. Weight loss, increased appetite, diarrhoea
5. Tachycardia, exertional dyspnoea, hyperdynamic circulation
6. Tiredness, irritability, nervousness
7. Fine tremor, hyperkinesia
8. Proximal muscle weakness with hyperactive reflexes
9. Occasionally, bone pain due to osteoporosis
10. In elderly patients, atrial fibrillation or cardiac failure

Extra-thyroid manifestations (possibly immunological)
11. Eye signs:
    Eyelid oedema
    Conjunctivitis
    Exophthalmos
    Lid retraction or lag
    Ophthalmoplegia (usually superior rectus)
12. Pretibial myxoedema
13. Thyroid acropachy (clubbing)
14. Vitiligo
15. Splenomegaly

MANAGEMENT OF THYROTOXICOSIS

1. Indications for thyroidectomy
   (i) Possible malignancy
   (ii) Pressure symptoms
   (iii) Retrosternal goitre
   (iv) Large goitre
   (v) Refusal or failure of medical treatment
   (vi) Hypersensitivity to antithyroid drugs
Patient must first be made euthyroid to avoid thyroid 'storm'

2. Indications for medical treatment
   (i) Young patients
   (ii) Pregnancy
   (iii) Mild hyperthyroidism with small goitre
   (iv) Patients unsuitable for surgery

3. Indications for radioiodine therapy
   (i) Relapse after thyroidectomy
   (ii) Patients over age 45
   (iii) Toxic adenomas
Subsequent hypothyroidism is common (about 40% at 10 years)

THE PARATHYROIDS
HYPERPARATHYROIDISM
CAUSES
1. **Primary**
   (i) Adenoma (single or multiple) (85%)
   (ii) Hyperplasia
   (iii) Carcinoma

2. **Secondary**
   Hyperplasia due to chronic renal failure, osteomalacia or rickets

3. **Tertiary**
   A complication of secondary hyperparathyroidism in which autonomous hyperparathyroidism develops

CLINICAL FEATURES
('Bones, stones, abdominal groans and psychic moans')

1. **Due to hypercalcaemia**
   (i) Anorexia, nausea and vomiting
   (ii) Constipation
   (iii) Polydipsia and polyuria
   (iv) Lethargy and depression, progressing to coma and convulsions

2. **Metastatic calcification**
   (i) Renal calculi
   (ii) Nephrocalcinosis
   (iii) Conjunctival deposits and keratopathy

3. **Bone resorption**
   (i) Pain and deformity
   (ii) Pathological fractures

4. **Rarely**
   Peptic ulcer, pancreatitis, pseudo-gout

HYPOPARATHYROIDISM
CAUSES
1. Postoperative (e.g. thyroidectomy)
2. Idiopathic (possibly autoimmune)
3. Neonatal (transient, but dangerous)

CLINICAL FEATURES

1. Due to hypocalcaemia
   (i) Tetany (paraesthesiae, stridor, cramps, hyperreflexia)
       Trousseau's and Chvostek's signs are present
   (ii) Convulsions (especially in children)
   (iii) Cataracts

2. In idiopathic hypoparathyroidism
   (i) Mental subnormality
   (ii) Dry skin, sparse hair, poor teeth, nail dystrophy often with
        candidosis
   (iii) Papilloedema and calcified basal ganglia (mimics brain
        tumour)
   (iv) Other autoimmune disorders, e.g. hypoadrenalism,
        pernicious anaemia

THE ADRENALS
CUSHING'S SYNDROME
CAUSES OF CUSHING'S SYNDROME

1. Iatrogenic (prednisolone or ACTH)
2. Alcoholism (pseudo-Cushing's)
3. Cushing's disease (pituitary-dependent adrenal hyperplasia)
4. Adrenal carcinoma or adenoma
5. Ectopic ACTH (e.g. small cell bronchial cancer)

CLINICAL FEATURES

1. Obesity of trunk and face with 'buffalo hump'
2. Hypertension
3. Skin changes:
   (i) Striae
   (ii) Bruising
   (iii) Hirsutism
   (iv) Pigmentation
4. Osteoporosis
5. Proximal myopathy
6. Menstrual disturbances
7. Neurosis or psychosis
8. Facial plethora due to polycythaemia

LABORATORY FEATURES

1. Increased plasma 11-hydroxycorticosteroids ('cortisol')
   Normal values:

9 a.m.	12 midnight
190–690 nmol/l	80–190 nmol/l
(7–25 µg/100 ml)	(3–7 µg/100 ml)

Loss of diurnal rhythm occurs early in Cushing's syndrome (i.e. midnight samples give increased value)
2. Polycythaemia with leukocytosis and eosinophil decrease
3. Hypokalaemia, with sodium in upper normal range
4. 'Diabetic' glucose tolerance test
5. 24 hour urinary 'free 11-hydroxycorticosteroids' increased

Low dosage dexamethasone (0.5 mg q.d.s. for 2 days) causes little suppression in Cushing's syndrome
High dosage dexamethasone (2 mg q.d.s. for 2 days) causes suppression in adrenal hyperplasia, but has little or no effect in adrenal adenoma or carcinoma, or ectopic ACTH secretion due to extra-adrenal carcinoma

HAZARDS OF SYSTEMIC GLUCOCORTICOID THERAPY

1. Growth retardation in children
2. Cushingoid facies, buffalo hump
3. Adrenal suppression and atrophy
4. Weight gain, sodium and water retention, potassium depletion
5. Hypertension
6. Hyperglycaemia
7. Hyperlipidaemia
8. Infections, especially viral, TB and fungal
9. Osteoporosis, aseptic bone necrosis, ruptured Achilles tendon
10. Gastrointestinal
    Dyspepsia
    Peptic ulcer and perforation
    Pancreatitis
11. CNS
    Euphoria
    Psychosis
    Increased intracranial pressure
    Increased tendency to epilepsy
12. Skin changes
    Thinning, striae and easy bruising
    Poor wound healing, enlargement of venous leg ulcers
    Acne
    Hypertrichosis
13. Myopathy or muscle atrophy
14. Cataracts, and raised intra-ocular pressure
15. Amenorrhoea or premature menopause
16. Teratogenicity (fetal cleft palate)
17. 'Rebound' of disease on reduction of dosage

CAUSES OF HYPOADRENALISM

ACUTE

1. Stress occurring in patients with chronic hypoadrenalism
2. Septicaemia, especially meningococcal (Waterhouse–Friedrichsen)
3. Surgical adrenalectomy
4. Abrupt withdrawal of steroid therapy
5. Pituitary necrosis (e.g. Sheehan's)

CHRONIC

Primary
1. Autoimmune adrenalitis (Addison's)
2. TB
3. Metastatic cancer deposits occur commonly, but rarely cause hypoadrenalism

Secondary (ACTH deficiency)
1. Pituitary or hypothalamic disease
2. Prolonged corticosteroid therapy

CLINICAL FEATURES OF CHRONIC HYPOADRENALISM

1. Pigmentation, especially in exposed skin, mouth, areolae, palmar creases, pressure areas and scars (except in hypopituitarism)
2. Debility and tiredness
3. Nausea, vomiting, weight loss, abdominal pain, diarrhoea
4. Hypotension, with low-volume pulse
5. Hypoglycaemia, especially reactive after a meal
6. Loss of body hair in women
7. Depression
8. May be associated autoimmune disorder, e.g. vitiligo

LABORATORY FEATURES OF HYPOADRENALISM

1. Plasma 11-hydroxycorticosteroids may be normal or low, but fail to respond adequately to 250 µg Synacthen i.m. (should rise by more than 193 nmol/l (7 µg/100 ml) at 30 minutes)
2. Low plasma sodium and chloride, with raised potassium and urea
3. Low voltage ECG with flat T waves
4. Low blood sugar, especially after fasting

DIABETES MELLITUS

CAUSES OF DIABETES MELLITUS

1. Idiopathic
   (i) Insulin-dependent ('juvenile')
   (ii) Non-insulin-dependent ('maturity onset')
2. Drug-induced
   Glucocorticoids, thiazides, diazoxide
3. Pancreatic disease
   Pancreatitis, cancer, haemochromatosis, glucagonoma, cystic fibrosis
4. Other metabolic disease
   Acromegaly, phaeochromocytoma, Cushing's, thyrotoxicosis
5. Genetic syndromes
   Glycogen storage disease, Down's syndrome, etc.

DIFFERENCES BETWEEN THE 2 MAIN TYPES OF DIABETES MELLITUS

'Juvenile'	*'Maturity onset'*
1. Thin	Obese
2. Young	Middle-aged or elderly
3. Tendency to ketosis	Resistant to ketosis
4. Low insulin secretion	Normal or increased insulin secretion
5. Sensitive to insulin	Insulin resistant
6. Require treatment with insulin	Respond to diet, and oral hypoglycaemic drugs
7. HLA-associated (DR3 and 4)	No association
8. Siblings rarely affected	Siblings often affected

DIFFERENCES BETWEEN 'DIABETIC' AND HYPOGLYCAEMIC COMA

Ketoacidaemic coma	*Hypoglycaemic coma*
1. Preceded by infection or insulin underdosage	Preceded by exercise, missed meal or insulin overdosage
2. Onset over hours or days	Onset in minutes
3. Deep rapid breathing	Stertorous breathing
4. Dehydration	Normal hydration
5. Sweating absent	Sweating marked
6. CNS changes unusual	CNS changes common, especially Babinski response
7. Urine — usually glycosuria and ketonuria	Urine not helpful

COMPLICATIONS OF DIABETES MELLITUS

1. **Ocular**
   (i) Blurred vision due to fluctuations in blood sugar

(ii) Cataracts
(iii) Retinopathy (see p. 94)
(iv) Rubeosis iridis (new blood vessels over iris) — may cause glaucoma

2. Neurological
(i) Peripheral neuropathy (early sign is loss of ankle jerks and malleolar vibration sense)
(ii) Mononeuritis multiplex (neuropathy of several peripheral or cranial nerves; often asymmetrical)
(iii) Autonomic neuropathy:
    a. Diarrhoea
    b. Postural hypotension
    c. Impotence
    d. Abnormal sweating
    e. Dependent oedema

3. Renal
(i) Pyelonephritis, sometimes with papillary necrosis
(ii) Glomerulonephritis
    a. Kimmelstiel–Wilson (eosinophilic nodules in glomerular tuft)
    b. Proliferative, with sclerosed basement membrane
(iii) Atherosclerosis and hypertensive vascular changes

4. Vascular
Occlusion by atheroma (large vessels) or endarteritis (small vessels) may cause ischaemia of feet, myocardium, brain or kidneys

5. Dermatological
(i) Fat atrophy or hypertrophy at insulin injection sites
(ii) Ulcers due to neuropathy or ischaemia
(iii) Infections, especially furuncles and candidosis
(iv) Pigmented scars over shins ('diabetic dermopathy')
(v) Xanthomata
(vi) Necrobiosis lipoidica

6. Systemic infections
Incidence of TB and deep mycoses is increased

CAUSES OF SHORT STATURE

1. 'CONSTITUTIONAL'
Racial, familial or sporadic

2. NUTRITIONAL
(i) Starvation

(ii) Malabsorption
(iii) Protein loss

3. CHROMOSOMAL DEFECTS

(i) Trisomies, e.g. Down's
(ii) Turner's

4. SKELETAL DEFECTS

(i)   Rickets
(ii) Achondroplasia
(iii) Gargoylism (Hurler's)

5. CHRONIC SYSTEMIC DISEASE

(i)   Cyanotic congenital heart disease
(ii)   Renal failure
(iii) Hepatic failure
(iv)   Pulmonary disease
(v)   Anaemia
(vi)   Infections, e.g. TB
(vii) Long-term steroid therapy (e.g. for asthma)

6. ENDOCRINE DISEASE

(i)   Sexual precocity
(ii) Hypopituitarism
(iii) Hypothyroidism
(iv) Congenital adrenal hyperplasia

7. MISCELLANEOUS RARE DISEASES

Diseases of unknown cause, e.g. progeria

CAUSES OF GYNAECOMASTIA

1. Neonatal, or normal puberty
2. Cirrhosis
3. Malignancy
4. Testicular or adrenal tumours
5. Drugs
    (i)   Oestrogens
    (ii) Cyproterone acetate
    (iii) Spironolactone
    (iv) Cimetidine
    (v)   Methyldopa
    (vi) Digoxin
6. Klinefelter's syndrome (XXY)

CAUSES OF GALACTORRHOEA

1. Physiological (postpartum or neonatal)
2. Prolactin-secreting pituitary tumour
3. Ectopic prolactin, e.g. bronchial Ca
4. Drugs
   - (i) Phenothiazines
   - (ii) Oral contraceptives
   - (iii) Methyldopa

SIDE-EFFECTS OF ORAL CONTRACEPTIVES

1. SYMPTOMS DUE TO OESTROGENS

Fluid retention, weight gain
Nausea and vomiting
Headache
Tiredness and irritability
Venous hypertension in legs
Increased menstrual loss

2. SYMPTOMS DUE TO PROGESTOGENS

Depression
Acne
Decreased libido, dry vagina
Muscle cramps
Breast discomfort
Reduced menstrual loss

3. GYNAECOLOGICAL

Amenorrhoea on contraceptive withdrawal
Cervical erosion
Vaginal candidiasis
Increase in size of fibroids

4. ENDOCRINE AND METABOLIC

Abnormal carbohydrate tolerance
Increased plasma triglycerides and cholesterol
Abnormal liver function tests
Plasma protein changes, e.g. increased transferrin
Increased thyroxine and plasma cortisol
Rarely:
   Hypertension
   Chloasma
   Galactorrhoea
   Gallstones

5. THROMBOEMBOLIC EFFECTS

Increased risk of thrombosis (e.g. coronary, cerebral) or embolism (e.g. pulmonary) due to increased clotting factors and platelet stickiness

CONTRA-INDICATIONS TO OESTROGENIC ORAL CONTRACEPTIVES

1. Pregnancy
2. Hepatic disease
3. Breast or cervical carcinoma
4. History of thrombosis or embolism
5. Care is required in patients with a history of epilepsy, arterial disease, hypertension, varicose veins, oedema, diabetes mellitus, prolactinoma, gallstones, migraine or fibroids. Women over age 35 are at increased risk of thromboembolic disease (esp. smokers)

OSTEOPOROSIS

A reduction in bone mass below the normal expected for the age and sex of the patient. Histologically the trabecular bone is reduced, and the mineral–matrix ratio is approximately normal

COMMON CAUSES

1. Old age
2. Immobilization
3. Glucocorticoid therapy (or Cushing's disease)
4. Sex hormone deficiency, e.g. premature menopause, Turner's syndrome
5. Cigarette smoking
6. Rheumatoid arthritis causes localized osteoporosis

OSTEOMALACIA

A reduction in the mineral–matrix ratio, although the total bone mass may be normal, decreased or even increased

CAUSES

1. Deficiency of cholecalciferol (vitamin D)

   (i) Inadequate diet, possibly aggravated by pregnancy or lack of UV radiation
  (ii) Malabsorption
 (iii) Phenytoin
2. Chronic renal failure
3. Hepatic disease (disturbed vitamin D metabolism)

Causes of hypercalcaemia
1. Hyperparathyroidism
2. Malignancy with or without metastases
3. Myelomatosis (rarely lymphoma or leukaemia)
4. Vit. D sensitivity, especially sarcoidosis
5. Vit. D excess
6. Milk–alkali syndrome

Causes of hypocalcaemia
1. Hypoparathyroidism
   (i) Post-thyroidectomy
  (ii) Idiopathic (sometimes with hypoadrenalism and candidosis)
2. Deficiency of cholecalciferol
3. Malabsorption
4. Chronic renal failure or Fanconi syndrome
5. Hypoalbuminaemia

PAGET'S DISEASE

CLINICAL FEATURES

1. Often asymptomatic. Incidence increases with age
2. Bone deformity
   (i) Enlarged skull
  (ii) Sabre tibia
 (iii) Long bone fractures
3. Nerve entrapment
   (i) Deafness
  (ii) Basilar invagination
 (iii) Cervical spondylosis
4. High output cardiac failure
5. Increased incidence of bone sarcoma

10. Renal disease

CLASSICAL PRESENTATIONS OF RENAL DISEASE

1. Haematuria alone
2. Proteinuria alone
3. Nephrotic syndrome (severe proteinuria, hypoalbuminaemia, peripheral oedema and often hyperlipidaemia)
4. Nephritic syndrome (haematuria, hypertension and peripheral oedema)
5. Acute renal failure (oliguria with acute uraemia)
6. Chronic renal failure (polyuria with insidious uraemia)

Renal disease which affects the glomeruli is called glomerulonephritis, and this is classified by the pathology shown on renal biopsy (p. 132). Many diseases can cause more than one of the above presentations. Thus membranous glomerulonephritis usually causes the nephrotic syndrome, but it can occasionally present as acute or chronic renal failure.

RENAL FAILURE

CAUSES OF ACUTE RENAL FAILURE

(A) Prerenal
1. Loss of blood, plasma or water and electrolytes
2. Hypotension with normal blood volume, e.g. myocardial infarct or septicaemic shock

(B) Renal
1. Acute-on-chronic failure, precipitated by renal infection or dehydration
2. Acute 'tubular necrosis' (or rarely cortical necrosis)
   - (i) Sustained hypotension
   - (ii) Obstetric causes, e.g. abortion or antepartum haemorrhage
   - (iii) Septicaemia (especially Gram-negative)
   - (iv) Free circulating haemoglobin
   - (v) Extensive tissue damage
   - (vi) Drugs and toxins, e.g. heavy metals, carbon tetrachloride, NSAID
3. Primary renal disease
   - (i) Acute glomerulonephritis

    (ii) Fulminating pyelonephritis
    (iii) Acute 'collagen–vascular disease'
4. Hepato-renal syndromes (including Weil's disease)
5. Vascular
    (i) Arterial — thrombosis, embolism, trauma
    (ii) Venous — thrombosis

(C) Postrenal
Obstruction in urinary tract (p. 137)

CAUSES OF CHRONIC RENAL FAILURE

1. Glomerulonephritis
2. Pyelonephritis or TB
3. Hypertension
4. Collagen–vascular disease, especially SLE and PAN
5. Metabolic
    (i) Diabetes mellitus
    (ii) Gout
    (iii) Chronic analgesic ingestion
    (iv) Amyloidosis
    (v) Hypercalcaemia
6. Obstruction in renal tract
7. Myeloma
8. Schistosomiasis (rare in UK)
9. Congenital
    (i) Polycystic kidney
    (ii) Tubular acidosis
    (iii) Fanconi syndrome

CLINICAL FEATURES OF SEVERE CHRONIC RENAL FAILURE

1. DERMATOLOGICAL

    (i) Pruritus
    (ii) Pallor
    (iii) Pigmentation
    (iv) Petechiae
    (v) White nails
    (vi) Rarely 'urea frost'

2. NEUROLOGICAL

    (i) Mental changes (confusion, paranoia, etc.)
    (ii) Apathy and weakness
    (iii) Muscle twitching and seizures
    (iv) Coma in terminal cases
    (v) Peripheral neuropathy in chronic undialysed cases

3. CARDIOVASCULAR

- (i) Pericarditis (may be tamponade)
- (ii) Cardiac failure due to salt and water overload
- (iii) Hypertension with retinopathy
- (iv) Arrhythmia (due to hyperkalaemia)

4. GASTROINTESTINAL

- (i) Dry mouth, foetor, may be parotitis
- (ii) Anorexia, nausea and vomiting
- (iii) Hiccups
- (iv) GI tract ulceration and bleeding

5. GENITOURINARY

- (i) In acute renal failure — oliguria (< 300 ml/24 h)
- (ii) In chronic renal failure — polyuria with fixed urinary specific gravity (1.010)

6. RESPIRATORY

- (i) Hyperventilation due to acidosis
- (ii) Pleural effusion

7. HAEMATOLOGICAL

- (i) Anaemia due to:
  - GI bleeding
  - Haemolysis
  - Dietary restrictions
  - Erythropoietin deficiency
- (ii) Bleeding tendency due to platelet dysfunction
- (iii) Susceptibility to secondary infection

8. DEFECTS IN BONE AND CALCIUM METABOLISM

- (i) Osteomalacia ('renal rickets' in children)
- (ii) Secondary or tertiary hyperparathyroidism (osteitis fibrosa cystica)
- (iii) Patchy osteosclerosis
- (iv) Occasionally osteoporosis
- (v) Occasionally metastatic calcification of muscles, blood vessels and conjunctivae

FACTORS WHICH MAY PRECIPITATE 'URAEMIA'

1. Fluid and electrolyte imbalance
2. Infection, systemic or urinary

3. Increased protein ingestion
4. Obstruction of renal tract
5. Catabolic or nephrotoxic drugs (e.g. tetracycline)
6. Congestive cardiac failure
7. Gastrointestinal haemorrhage or surgery

GLOMERULONEPHRITIS

This may be: *Focal* — some glomeruli are affected
     or *Diffuse* — all glomeruli are affected

        Segmental — part of a glomerulus is affected
     or *Global* — all of a glomerulus is affected

  Thus, in focal segmental glomerulonephritis, parts of some glomeruli are affected

CLASSIFICATION OF GLOMERULONEPHRITIS

1. Minimal change
No change on light microscopy but EM shows loss of podocytes
Typically affects children but may be due to NSAIDs in adults
Produces acute nephrotic syndrome, but good prognosis

2. IgA disease (*Berger's disease*)
Similar to Henoch–Schönlein purpura, with which it may overlap
Typically causes haematuria in young men
20% develop renal failure over 15 years

3. Proliferative
Traditionally follows Group A streptococcal infection, but now not usually associated in UK. Low C3 during the acute attack. Good prognosis

4. Membranous
Due to
Malaria
Malignancy (e.g. bronchial cancer)
Hepatitis **B**
Rheumatoid **A**rthritis (and penicillamine or gold therapy for RA)
SLE
Mnemonic: MeMBRAnouS

Prognosis: 1/3 improve, 1/3 stay the same, 1/3 progress
Commonest form of de novo glomerulonephritis in renal allografts

5. Mesangiocapillary (types I and II)
C3 usually low
Type II is associated with partial lipoatrophy and with C3
nephritic factor

6. Focal
Associated with **WE**gener's granulomatosis, **SLE**, **E**ndocarditis,
Polyarteritis nodosa, **HE**noch–Schönlein purpura
Mnemonic: WE SLEEP HEre

7. Rapidly progressive (*crescentic*)
Associated with **W**egener's granulomatosis, **H**enoch–Schönlein
purpura, **A**ntiglomerular basement membrane
(Goodpasture's), **M**icroscopic polyangiitis, **I**mmune complex
disease
Mnemonic: WHAMI

8. Focal segmental glomerulosclerosis
Sometimes idiopathic, particularly in children, but in adults
usually secondary to other forms of glomerulonephritis or
other renal disease such as pyelonephritis or severe
hypertension

CAUSES OF NEPHROTIC SYNDROME

1. Glomerulonephritis accounts for 80% (usually membranous in
   adults, minimal change in children)
2. Metabolic
   (i) Diabetes mellitus
   (ii) Amyloidosis
   (iii) Myelomatosis
3. SLE
4. Drugs — mercurials, penicillamine, troxidone
5. Renal vein thrombosis

CAUSES OF LARGE KIDNEY (OR KIDNEYS)

1. Cystic kidneys
2. Hydronephrosis or pyonephrosis
3. Hypernephroma
4. Hypertrophy following contralateral nephrectomy or failure
5. Nephrotic syndrome
   Also consider the possibility of perirenal haematoma

TYPES OF RENAL TUBULAR DYSFUNCTION

1. RENAL DISEASE AFFECTING MEDULLA
   e.g. pyelonephritis. Impairment of urinary concentration,
   acidification and electrolyte reabsorption

2. RENAL GLYCOSURIA (benign)

3. 'VITAMIN D RESISTANT RICKETS'

Inability to reabsorb phosphate

4. IDIOPATHIC HYPERCALCIURIA

Inability to reabsorb calcium

5. RENAL TUBULAR ACIDOSIS (Type I — distal tubules)

Inability to acidify the urine causes metabolic acidosis. Less calcium is bound to protein and calcium filtration is increased, leading to nephrocalcinosis and renal stones

6. RENAL TUBULAR ACIDOSIS (Type 2 — proximal tubules)

Occurs as part of Fanconi syndrome, with defective reabsorption of glucose, amino acids and phosphate (GAP) Hyperchloraemic acidosis occurs, but no nephrocalcinosis May also be due to toxins (lead, mercury, outdated tetracycline), kidney transplant or cystinosis

7. CYSTINURIA

Defect in reabsorption of cystine, ornithine, arginine and lysine (COAL)
Cystine stones form

8. NEPHROGENIC DIABETES INSIPIDUS

Impaired response to ADH

ACID–BASE BALANCE

These headings reflect changes in extracellular fluid only, e.g. in metabolic alkalosis there is an associated intracellular acidosis

1. RESPIRATORY ACIDOSIS (low pH, high CO_2 content)

Any cause of hypoventilation (p. 43)

2. RESPIRATORY ALKALOSIS (high pH, low CO_2 content)

Any cause of hyperventilation (e.g. aspirin overdose or anxiety)

3. METABOLIC ACIDOSIS (low pH, low CO_2 content)

Causes

(i) **Ingestion of acidic compounds**
Ammonium chloride, salicylates, etc.

(ii) **Metabolic overproduction of acids**
Ketosis, e.g. starvation, diabetes mellitus
Lactic acidosis

(iii) **Intestinal loss of base**
Diarrhoea
Fistulae

(iv) **Renal failure: renal tubular acidosis**

4. METABOLIC ALKALOSIS (high pH, high CO_2 content)

Causes
Ingestion of alkali, e.g. $NaHCO_3$, for indigestion
Vomiting, or gastric aspiration
Hypokalaemia

CAUSES OF HYPOKALAEMIA

1. **Increased renal loss**
   (i) Diuresis
       Drugs, e.g. thiazides
       Diabetes mellitus
   (ii) Minerolocorticoid excess, e.g. primary aldosteronism
       (Conn's tumour) and Cushing's disease
   (iii) Primary renal disease, e.g. chronic pyelonephritis

2. **Increased intestinal loss**
   e.g. diarrhoea, vomiting
   Consider purgative abuse

3. **Decreased intake**
   Dietary lack (especially in alcoholism, or during protein
   anabolism in convalescence, or following prolonged i.v. fluids)
   Malabsorption

CLINICAL FEATURES OF POTASSIUM DEPLETION

1. Muscle weakness
2. Apathy, anorexia and confusion
3. Ileus
4. Increased cardiac excitability and digitalis toxicity
5. Thirst and polyuria

CAUSES OF HYPONATRAEMIA

1. **Excessive water intake**
   Oral (polydipsia) or intravenous

2. **Excessive water retention**
   Inappropriate ADH secretion

3. **Inadequate sodium intake** (rare)

4. **Inadequate sodium retention**
   - (i) Vomiting, diarrhoea, ileus, fistula, drainage of ascites
   - (ii) Hypoadrenalism
   - (iii) Renal loss
   - (iv) Skin loss
     - a. Excessive sweating
     - b. Cystic fibrosis
     - c. Burns

CAUSES OF POLYURIA

1. Chronic renal failure
2. Diabetes mellitus
3. Diuretic drugs
4. Compulsive water drinking
5. Diabetes insipidus
   - (i) Pituitary (deficiency of ADH)
   - (ii) Nephrogenic (no response to ADH)
6. Potassium depletion
7. Hypercalcaemia

CAUSES OF PROTEINURIA

1. Contamination (semen, prostatic or vaginal secretion)
2. Postural (orthostatic)
3. Renal disease
   - (i) Glomerulonephritis, especially nephrotic syndrome
   - (ii) Pyelonephritis
   - (iii) Obstructive nephropathy
   - (iv) Malignant hypertension
   - (v) Tuberculosis
4. Disease of renal tract, e.g. cystitis
5. May be slight albuminuria in fever or congestive heart failure
6. Multiple myeloma (Bence Jones protein)

CAUSES OF HAEMATURIA

(A) KIDNEY LESIONS

1. Glomerulonephritis, pyelonephritis, TB
2. Trauma

3. Anticoagulant overdose, bleeding diathesis
4. Hypernephroma
5. Renal infarct (including polyarteritis nodosa)
6. Polycystic kidney
7. Bacterial endocarditis

(B) RENAL TRACT LESIONS

1. Papillary tumour of bladder
2. Acute cystitis (including cyclophosphamide toxicity)
3. Calculi
4. Prostatic lesions:
    Hypertrophy
    Cancer
    Prostatitis
5. Urethral inflammation or trauma
6. TB (now rare in UK)
7. Schistosomiasis (rare in UK)

CAUSES OF 'STERILE' PYURIA

1. Renal TB
2. Analgesic nephropathy
3. Renal calculi
4. Urinary infection treated with chemotherapy
5. Non-specific urethritis

CAUSES OF 'DARK COLOURED' URINE

1. Concentration
2. Bile
3. Blood, haemoglobinuria and myoglobinuria
4. Methaemoglobinuria
5. Porphyria
6. Alkaptonuria
7. Melaninuria
8. Beetroot, dyes in sweets, drugs (e.g. rifampicin), etc.

CAUSES OF URINARY TRACT OBSTRUCTION

1. Stone
2. Stricture (post-op or inflammatory)
3. Stenosis (congenital)   } occur throughout
4. Neoplasm   the urinary tract
5. Clot
6. Neuromuscular incoordination
7. Retroperitoneal fibrosis   } ureter
8. Spread of cancer from pelvic organs

9. Prostatic enlargement or cancer
10. Retroverted gravid uterus   } bladder neck
11. Trauma of labour
12. Congenital valves   } urethra
13. Phimosis or paraphimosis

Common causes of acute retention in adults are:

Males
1. Post-operative retention
2. Prostatic lesions

3. Urethral stricture

Females
1. Trauma of labour
2. Pressure from uterus (fetus or fibroid)
3. Hysteria

Remember that retention may also be due to anticholinergic drugs or a neurological lesion such as multiple sclerosis or cord compression

URINARY CALCULI

FACTORS WHICH PREDISPOSE TO URINARY CALCULI

1. Metabolic abnormalities (q.v.)
2. Urinary tract infections, e.g. Proteus
3. Urinary tract stasis
4. Foreign bodies in urinary tract
5. Geographical factors (e.g. hot, dry climate, hard water)

METABOLIC CAUSES OF URINARY CALCULI

CALCIUM STONES (composed of calcium oxalate, phosphate or both)

1. Hypercalciuria (on normal diet, > 300 mg/24 h in male or > 250 mg/24 h in female)
    (i) Idiopathic hypercalciuria
    (ii) Hyperparathyroidism
    (iii) Vitamin D excess
    (iv) Sarcoidosis
    (v) Milk–alkali syndrome
    (vi) Renal tubular acidosis
    (vii) Malignancy
    (viii) Immobilization
    (ix) Cushing's syndrome
2. Alkaline urine
3. Oxaluria

URIC ACID STONES

Primary or secondary gout
Uricosuric drugs

CYSTINE STONES

Cystinuria
Fanconi syndrome with cystinosis

XANTHINE STONES

Xanthinuria

RENAL STONES

Radio-opaque
Calcium (80%)
Mg ammonium phosphate (10%)
Cystine (2%)

Non-opaque
Uric acid (5%)
Xanthine (1%)

NEUROLOGICAL CONTROL OF BLADDER FUNCTION

Normal bladder capacity is 300–400 ml and larger volumes should
stimulate the desire to micturate. Afferent fibres travel via
parasympathetic nerves to spinal 'micturition centre' (S 2, 3, 4)
and bladder contraction is initiated by parasympathetic efferents.
The spinal 'micturition centre' is normally inhibited by higher
motor centres, which bombard it with facilitatory impulses when
micturition begins, so that the bladder empties completely

TYPES OF DYSFUNCTION

1. LACK OF NORMAL INHIBITION

   Frequency with small volumes
   Occurs in anxiety, cold weather, etc.

2. ATONIC BLADDER

   Distended bladder with overflow, but no desire to micturate
   Occurs with sensory neuropathy, e.g. diabetes mellitus, tabes
   dorsalis

3. AUTOMATIC BLADDER

   Bladder empties partially when volume of about 250 ml is
   reached, but without desire to micturate
   Occurs with cord section above S 2, 3, 4

4. AUTONOMOUS BLADDER

   Large residual urine volume, with weak uncoordinated bladder
   contractions but no desire to micturate. Occurs with LMN cord
   lesions at S 2, 3, 4 level

Unilateral neurological lesions may cause either frequency with small volumes or a large hypotonic bladder with residual urine after micturition

RENAL CLEARANCE

The number of ml of plasma which contains the amount of a substance excreted in the urine in one minute is the renal clearance of that substance, i.e. $C = UV/PT$ ml
where U = concentration of substance in urine
$\qquad V$ = volume of urine collected in time T
$\qquad P$ = concentration of substance in plasma

Creatinine clearance gives a more accurate measure of renal function than the plasma urea

11. Rheumatology

PATTERNS OF POLYARTHROPATHY
PRIMARY OSTEOARTHROSIS
Symmetrical, affecting many joints
1. Knees
2. Great toes and thumbs: MP joints
3. Fingers: terminal IP joints
4. Acromioclavicular joints
5. Small joints of spine

SECONDARY OSTEOARTHROSIS
Asymmetrical, affecting weight-bearing joints
1. Knees
2. Hip
3. Intervertebral discs

RHEUMATOID ARTHRITIS
Usually symmetrical, intermittent and inflamed
1. Hands: intercarpal joints, MP joints and proximal IP joints
2. Feet: tarsal and lateral MP joints
3. Knees
4. Small joints of cervical spine and subacromial bursae

ANKYLOSING SPONDYLITIS
1. Spine and both sacroiliac joints
2. Knees, shoulders, wrists

PSORIASIS
1. Hands, terminal IP joints (look for nail pits)
2. Sacroiliac joints
3. 'Rheumatoid' pattern
4. Asymmetrical oligoarthritis (e.g. knee)
5. Arthritis mutilans

REITER'S DISEASE
1. Ankles and all joints of feet

2. Knees
3. Hips, sacroiliac joints and spine

X-RAY CHANGES OF OSTEOARTHROSIS

1. Joint space narrowing
2. Subarticular sclerosis
3. Osteophytes
4. Bone cysts

JOINT COMPLICATIONS OF RHEUMATOID ARTHRITIS

1. Deformity, subluxation, misalignment, swelling
2. Infection (septic arthritis)
3. Tendon rupture
4. Synovial sac protrusion and rupture (e.g. Baker's cyst)
5. Juxta-articular osteoporosis
6. Muscle atrophy secondary to disuse

EXTRA-ARTICULAR MANIFESTATIONS OF RHEUMATOID DISEASE

1. ANAEMIA

    (i) Fe deficiency (GI blood loss caused by drugs)
    (ii) Defective iron utilization (anaemia of chronic disorders)
    (iii) Marrow depression

2. PULMONARY

    (i) Pleuritis, effusions
    (ii) Nodules in lung or pleura
    (iii) Fibrosing alveolitis

3. CARDIAC

    (i) Pericarditis
    (ii) Nodules in myocardium

4. OCULAR

    (i) Scleritis, episcleritis
    (ii) Scleromalacia perforans
    (iii) Sicca syndrome (Sjögren's)

5. ARTERITIS

    (i) Digital ischaemia (may be Raynaud's)
    (ii) Nail fold lesions
    (iii) Leg ulcers
    (iv) Mesenteric ischaemia

6. PERIPHERAL NEUROPATHY (due to vasculitis)

7. ENTRAPMENT NEUROPATHY, e.g. spinal cord at cervical level from atlanto-axial subluxation, or carpal tunnel syndrome

8. FELTY'S SYNDROME (RA with leukopenia and splenomegaly)

9. LYMPHADENOPATHY

10. AMYLOIDOSIS

SERONEGATIVE SPONDYLOARTHRITIS (HLA-B27 ASSOCIATION)

Arthritis involving the spine but with consistent absence of rheumatoid factors from serum
1. Ankylosing spondylitis
2. Psoriatic arthritis
3. Enteropathic arthritis (Crohn's, ulcerative colitis, Whipple's, enteric infection, intestinal bypass for obesity)
4. Reiter's disease

FEATURES OF ANKYLOSING SPONDYLITIS

1. Ankylosis/arthritis of spine (bamboo spine)
2. Anterior uveitis
3. Arrhythmia
4. Aortic regurgitation
5. Apical pulmonary fibrosis

(*N.B.* 5 **A**s)

CAUSES OF LUMBAR BACKACHE

1. MECHANICAL
    (i) Musculotendinous and ligament strain
    (ii) Prolapsed intervertebral disc
    (iii) Spondylosis and spondylolisthesis
    (iv) Spinal fracture
        a. Major trauma
        b. Crush fracture in osteoporosis
        c. Stress fracture of transverse process due to muscular effort

2. DEGENERATIVE OR METABOLIC

   (i) Osteoarthrosis
   (ii) Osteoporosis
   (iii) Osteomalacia

3. INFLAMMATORY

   (i) Infection, e.g. TB, pyogenic
   (ii) Seronegative spondyloarthritis (q.v.)

4. NEOPLASM

   (i) Usually metastatic malignancy
   (ii) Primary malignancy — Osteosarcoma
                              Myeloma
                              Lymphoma

5. REFERRED PAIN

   (i) Posterior duodenal ulcer
   (ii) Cancer of pancreas
   (iii) Renal colic
   (iv) Pelvic carcinoma
   (v) Dysmenorrhoea, labour pains

CAUSES OF A SINGLE HOT RED JOINT

1. Traumatic, e.g. sprained ankle
2. Septic arthritis
   May be secondary to penetrating injury, osteomyelitis, septicaemia, rheumatoid arthritis or osteoarthrosis
3. Gout or pseudo-gout (chondrocalcinosis or periarticular calcification)
4. Haemophilia
5. Gonococcal arthritis
6. Occasionally rheumatoid arthritis

CAUSES OF A TRANSIENT 'FLITTING' ARTHRITIS

1. Rheumatic fever
2. Henoch–Schönlein purpura
3. Serum sickness and drug reactions
4. SLE
5. Systemic infections
      (i) Gonococcal or meningococcal septicaemia
      (ii) Bacterial endocarditis
      (iii) Rubella

(iv) Infectious mononucleosis
(v) Infective hepatitis
(vi) Mycoplasma pneumonia
6. Reiter's disease
7. Occasionally, acute rheumatoid arthritis

CAUSES OF HYPERURICAEMIA

1. INCREASED PURINE SYNTHESIS

Primary gout (in 25% of cases)

2. DECREASED RENAL EXCRETION

(i) Primary gout (in 75% of cases)
(ii) Chronic renal failure
(iii) Drugs
Salicylates (in low dosage)
Uricosurics (in low dosage)
Thiazide diuretics
Alcohol

3. INCREASED TURNOVER OF PREFORMED PURINES

(i) Myeloproliferative disease and lymphoma (esp. after cytotoxic drugs)
(ii) Chronic haemolysis
(iii) Psoriasis

CLASSIFICATION OF VASCULITIS

No classification is completely satisfactory, since the clinical syndromes may overlap, and their pathogenesis is imperfectly understood

1. SYSTEMIC NECROTIZING VASCULITIS

(i) Polyarteritis nodosa
(ii) Churg–Strauss syndrome (with asthma and eosinophilia)
(iii) Wegener's granulomatosis (upper and lower respiratory tracts and kidneys)
(iv) Behçet's disease (with orogenital aphthous ulcers)

N.B. Antineutrophilic cytoplasmic antibodies:
cANCA is fairly sensitive for Wegener's
pANCA (perinuclear) is found in a broader range of vasculitides, including PAN

2. 'HYPERSENSITIVITY' VASCULITIS
(small vessel disease, often cutaneous with circulating immune complexes)
   - (i) Serum sickness is the classical example, but now rare
   - (ii) Drug allergy
   - (iii) Henoch–Schönlein purpura (affects skin, joints, GI tract and kidneys)
   - (iv) Infection (classically TB, e.g. Bazin's)
   - (v) Idiopathic cutaneous vasculitis (often nodular, on legs)
   - (vi) Malignancy, e.g. breast cancer

3. COLLAGEN VASCULAR DISEASE

   Rheumatoid, SLE, systemic sclerosis, dermatomyositis/polymyositis

4. LARGE VESSEL VASCULITIS

   Giant cell aortitis (e.g. Takayashu's)
   Temporal arteritis
   Kawasaki disease (usually young children, may be coronary arteritis)

5. THROMBOANGIITIS OBLITERANS
(Buerger's disease, occurs in smokers)

CLINICAL FEATURES OF POLYARTERITIS NODOSA (PAN)

Usually young or middle-aged men
1. Fever, malaise, weight loss
2. Gastrointestinal ischaemia
     Central abdominal pain
     Bleeding
3. Proteinuria and haematuria. Hypertension is common
4. Peripheral neuropathy, often painful
     Focal CNS lesions
5. Arthralgia and myalgia
6. Myocardial ischaemia
7. Skin lesions:
     Nodules
     Livedo reticularis
     Necrosis and ulceration

CLINICAL FEATURES OF SYSTEMIC LUPUS ERYTHEMATOSUS

Usually young or middle-aged women
1. Fever, malaise, weight loss

2. Arthralgia, flitting or episodic
3. Skin changes
    (i) Photosensitive rash, classically in butterfly distribution. May be erythematous, urticated or purpuric
    (ii) Alopecia
    (iii) Dilated nail fold capillaries
    (iv) Raynaud's phenomenon
4. Proteinuria, glomerulonephritis, nephrotic syndrome or hypertension
5. Lymphadenopathy
6. Myocarditis, endocarditis (Libman–Sacks), or pericarditis
7. Pleurisy with effusion, pneumonitis
8. Hepatomegaly and splenomegaly
9. Pancytopenia. May be haemolysis
10. Psychosis, neuropathy or epilepsy. May be retinal exudates
11. Gastrointestinal upsets (nausea, pain, diarrhoea, etc.)

RAYNAUD'S PHENOMENON

Paroxysmal digital ischaemia, which usually causes a characteristic sequence of colour changes (white, then blue, then red)

CAUSES

1. **Reflex vasoconstriction**
    (i) Raynaud's disease (idiopathic)
    (ii) Vibrating machinery

2. **Arterial occlusion**
    (i) Thoracic outlet syndromes
    (ii) Atheroma. Buerger's disease

3. **Collagen–vascular disease, especially systemic sclerosis and SLE**

4. **Increased blood viscosity**
    (i) Dysproteinaemias (macro- and cryoglobulinaemias)
    (ii) Polycythaemia, leukaemia

5. **Neurological disease,** especially syringomyelia or paralysis

12. Dermatology

PSORIASIS

DISTINCTIVE MORPHOLOGICAL TYPES

1. Nummular — discoid plaques, which may be confluent. Typically on extensor surfaces
2. Guttate — 'showers' of small lesions, often post-streptococcal
3. Erythrodermic — very widespread erythema, with exfoliation
4. Generalized pustular psoriasis
5. Pustular eruptions of the hands and feet

Atypical forms are common, e.g. follicular, intertriginous, etc.

'Napkin psoriasis' (psoriasiform lesions in infants) may be related to candida infection

ECZEMA

Eczema is a distinctive inflammatory response of the skin, characterized histologically by spongiosis (epidermal oedema) and clinically by clustered papulo-vesicles with erythema and scaling.
Many cases have a multifactorial aetiology

TYPES OF ECZEMA

(A) Exogenous
1. Primary irritant dermatitis, e.g. due to caustics, detergents or solvents
2. Allergic contact dermatitis, e.g. due to hypersensitivity to metals, rubber, medicaments, etc.
3. Infective dermatitis, e.g. around infected wounds or ulcers

(B) Endogenous
1. Atopic dermatitis (infantile eczema). Typically on flexor surfaces
2. Seborrhoeic dermatitis
3. Discoid eczema
4. Pompholyx — vesicles on palms or soles
5. Pityriasis alba — patches of scaly eczema which leave depigmented areas
6. Asteatotic eczema — due to excessive drying ('chapping')
7. Gravitational eczema — secondary to venous insufficiency

BLISTERING ERUPTIONS
COMMON CAUSES

1. Viral
    (i) Herpes simplex
    (ii) Herpes zoster — varicella
2. Impetigo
3. Scabies
4. Insect bites and papular urticaria
5. Bullous eczema and pompholyx
6. Drugs, e.g. barbiturate overdose, photosensitivity

UNCOMMON CAUSES

7. Erythema multiforme
8. Dermatitis herpetiformis
9. Pemphigoid   sub-epidermal
10. Porphyria cutanea tarda
11. Pemphigus group   intra-epidermal

Remember pemphigu**S** is **S**uperficial and pemphigoi**D** is **D**eeper

RARE CAUSES

12. Congenital
    (i)   Epidermolysis bullosa
    (ii) Ichthyosiform erythroderma
    (iii) Incontinentia pigmenti

CAUSES OF PHOTOSENSITIVITY (ENHANCED RESPONSE TO UV IRRADIATION)

1. Drugs, e.g. **t**olbutamide, **c**hlorpropamide, **p**henothiazines, **t**hiazides, **a**miodarone, **n**alidixic acid
    Mnemonic: TCP-TAN
2. Contact photosensitizers, e.g. tar, perfumes, soaps, etc.
3. Dermatoses, e.g. porphyria, polymorphic light eruption, lupus erythematosus
4. Decreased melanin in skin, e.g. albinism, vitiligo

CAUSES OF LEG ULCERS

1. Venous hypertension (90%)
2. Ischaemia
    (i) Atheroma
    (ii) Arteritis
3. Neuropathy
    (i) Diabetes mellitus

  (ii) Spina bifida
  (iii) Tabes dorsalis
  (iv) Leprosy (in endemic areas)
4. Rheumatoid arthritis — ulceration is multifactorial
5. Malignancy — usually squamous-cell skin carcinoma
6. Haemolytic anaemia, especially sickle-cell
7. Syphilitic gumma
8. Necrobiosis lipoidica (may be diabetic)
9. Pyoderma gangrenosum — often due to ulcerative colitis

Many leg ulcers have a multifactorial aetiology, e.g. ischaemia, anaemia, venous hypertension and infection

CAUSES OF ALOPECIA

1. Male-pattern baldness
2. Idiopathic diffuse alopecia of women — usually post-menopausal
3. 'Telogen effluvium' — loss of club hairs after febrile illness, surgery or parturition
4. Alopecia areata
5. Drugs:
     (i)   Cytotoxic agents
     (ii) Anticoagulants
     (iii) Dextran
     (iv) Oral contraceptives
6. Scalp infection:
     (i) Fungi
     (ii) Pyogenic bacteria
7. Systemic disease:
     (i)   Syphilis
     (ii) Hypothyroidism
     (iii) Fe deficiency
8. Traumatic:
     (i)   Traction from rollers
     (ii) Scalping injury
     (iii) Burns
     (iv) Excessive bleaching, perming, etc.
9. Dermatoses:
     (i)   Psoriasis
     (ii) Discoid lupus erythematosus
     (iii) Lichen planus
10. Congenital — many rare diseases, e.g. monilethrix

CAUSES OF HIRSUTISM

1. Idiopathic (including racial and familial variation)
2. Ovarian disease
     (i) Polycystic ovaries (common)
     (ii) Virilizing tumour (rare)

3. Adrenal hyperplasia or tumour
4. Obesity and hyperinsulinaemia
5. Prolactinoma
6. Androgenic drugs, e.g. methyltestosterone, anabolic steroids. (Other drugs such as minoxidil and diazoxide cause hypertrichosis rather than true hirsutism)

CAUSES OF DIFFUSE HYPERPIGMENTATION

1. Congenital (racial or familial)
2. Irradiation, esp. ultraviolet
3. Post-inflammatory, e.g. after erythroderma
4. Endocrine causes
   (i) Pregnancy, oestrogens
   (ii) Hypoadrenalism (due to MSH/beta-lipotrophin)
   (iii) Acromegaly
5. Miscellaneous systemic diseases
   (i) Cachexia (esp. TB or malignancy)
   (ii) Chronic renal failure
   (iii) Primary biliary cirrhosis
   (iv) Haemochromatosis
   (v) Malabsorption
6. Drugs, e.g. busulphan, chlorpromazine, ACTH, arsenic

SKIN DISEASES WHICH CAUSE SEVERE ITCHING

1. Parasites: scabies, pediculosis, flea bites
2. Eczema
3. Urticaria
4. Lichen planus
5. Lichen simplex chronicus
6. Dermatitis herpetiformis

SYSTEMIC CAUSES OF GENERALIZED PRURITUS

1. Obstructive jaundice (especially biliary cirrhosis)
2. Chronic renal failure
3. Lymphoma (especially Hodgkin's) or myeloproliferative disease (especially polycythaemia vera)
4. Carcinoma (especially bronchial)
5. Iron deficiency
6. Hypo- or hyperthyroidism
7. Drugs
   (i) Allergy
   (ii) Pharmacological, e.g. cocaine, morphine

N.B. a. Many women develop pruritus during pregnancy
     b. Scabies is easily missed in hygienic patients — remember to look for burrows in the fingerwebs, and examine the nipples or penis for typical papules

CAUSES OF GENERALIZED PALLOR

1. Vasoconstriction (cold, emotion, vasovagal, etc.)
2. Anaemia (including acute haemorrhage)
3. Diffuse hypomelanosis
   (i) Protection from UV radiation
   (ii) Albinism
   (iii) Phenylketonuria
   (iv) Hypopituitarism
   (v) Widespread vitiligo

CAUSES OF WHITE PATCHES ON THE SKIN (leukoderma)

1. *Congenital* (rare), e.g. tuberous sclerosis, partial albinism
2. *Post-inflammatory*, e.g. eczema, burns, discoid lupus erythematosus
3. *Infection*, e.g. leprosy, pityriasis versicolor
4. *Immunological*, e.g. vitiligo, halo naevus

ERYTHEMA

CAUSES OF PALMAR ERYTHEMA

1. Dermatoses, e.g. eczema or psoriasis
2. Increased oestrogens
   (i) Pregnancy
   (ii) Alcoholic cirrhosis
3. Rheumatoid arthritis
4. Shoulder-hand syndrome
5. Polycythaemia

CAUSES OF FACIAL FLUSHING

1. Heat and exertion
2. Psychological (blushing, anger)
3. Menopause
4. Rosacea
5. Food and drugs
   (i) Alcohol; marked in Mongoloid races, and in some diabetics taking chlorpropamide
   (ii) Peppers, chillies
   (iii) Nitrites, sodium monoglutamate, morphine, etc.
6. Carcinoid syndrome

SOME CAUSES OF A CIRCUMSCRIBED PATCH OF RED SCALY RASH

1. Psoriasis
2. Eczema

3. Fixed drug eruption
4. Fungus
5. Lichen simplex
6. Bowen's disease (squamous Ca in situ)
7. Discoid lupus erythematosus
8. Lupus vulgaris (a form of TB)

SOME CAUSES OF WIDESPREAD PATCHES OF RED SCALY RASH

1. Psoriasis
2. Eczema
3. Pityriasis rosea
4. Pityriasis versicolor
5. Secondary syphilis
6. Lichen planus
7. Fungus

CAUSES OF ERYTHRODERMA (inflammatory skin disease affecting more than 90% of body surface)

1. Eczema of various types (esp. atopic)
2. Psoriasis
3. Lymphoma or lymphatic leukaemia
4. Drugs, esp. gold or mercury
5. Idiopathic and rare congenital disorders

CAUSES OF ERYTHEMA NODOSUM (tender nodules on legs)

1. Sarcoidosis
2. Streptococcal infection
3. TB
4. Drugs, e.g. sulphonamides
5. Ulcerative colitis or Crohn's disease
6. Other infections, e.g.
   (i) Leprosy
   (ii) Systemic mycoses
   (iii) Toxoplasmosis
   (iv) Lymphogranuloma venereum

CAUSES OF ERYTHEMA MULTIFORME (often 'targets' on palms)

1. Infections, esp. herpes simplex, orf or mycoplasma
2. Drugs (many, esp. long-acting sulphonamides)
3. Idiopathic (recurrent forms may be due to occult herpes simplex)
4. Rarely collagen–vascular disease, pregnancy or malignancy

CAUSES OF PYODERMA GANGRENOSUM

1. Crohn's and other inflammatory bowel disorders (UC, etc.)
2. Rheumatoid and other inflammatory joint disorders
3. Idiopathic
4. Rarely dysproteinaemia or myeloproliferative disease (esp. leukaemia)

COMMON CAUSES OF A PIGMENTED PAPULE

1. Basal cell papilloma ('seborrhoeic wart')
2. Melanocytic naevus ('mole')
3. Malignant melanoma
4. Pigmented basal cell carcinoma
5. Dermatofibroma

FEATURES SUGGESTING MALIGNANT CHANGE IN A MOLE

Major features:
1. Change in *size* (esp. steady enlargement, though benign moles often enlarge at puberty and in pregnancy)
2. Change in *shape* (irregular outline may be important)
3. Change in *colour* (blotchy variation, or spread of pigment beyond margin may be important)

Minor features:
4. Diameter more than 7 mm
5. Inflammation
6. Ulceration or bleeding
7. Itch (though this is common in benign moles)

If diagnosis is uncertain obtain an expert opinion or excise for histology
   In malignant melanoma, the best indicator of prognosis is the Breslow thickness (vertical thickness on histology)

CAUSES OF XANTHOMA

1. Idiopathic, with normal blood lipids
2. Primary hyperlipidaemia, e.g. type 2 (hypercholesterolaemia)
3. Secondary hyperlipidaemia
    (i) Diabetes mellitus
    (ii) Hypothyroidism
    (iii) Chronic renal failure or nephrotic syndrome
    (iv) Cholestasis (esp. primary biliary cirrhosis)

   Other causes of hyperlipidaemia, less likely to produce xanthomas, include obesity, alcoholism, pancreatitis and drugs, e.g. isotretinoin

SKIN CHANGES ASSOCIATED WITH SYSTEMIC MALIGNANCY

1. GENETIC SYNDROMES PREDISPOSING TO MALIGNANCY

    e.g. neurofibromatosis (may develop glioma), familial tylosis (palmar keratoderma) with oesophageal carcinoma

2. SIGNS OF EXPOSURE TO A CARCINOGEN

    e.g.:
    (i) Nicotine staining of fingers
    (ii) Palmar keratoses due to arsenic

3. DIRECT INVOLVEMENT OF SKIN BY MALIGNANT CELLS

    (i) Direct spread from underlying cancer (especially breast)
    (ii) Cutaneous metastases
    (iii) Leukaemic or lymphomatous infiltrate

4. MISCELLANEOUS ENDOCRINE, METABOLIC AND IMMUNOLOGICAL EFFECTS

    (i) Pigmentation, pallor or pruritus
    (ii) Acanthosis nigricans
    (iii) Dermatomyositis
    (iv) Clubbing
    (v) Widespread viral infection (e.g. herpes) due to immune deficiency, etc.

NAIL CHANGES DUE TO SYSTEMIC DISEASE

ABNORMAL MORPHOLOGY

1. Clubbing (p. 46)
2. Koilonychia (iron deficiency)
3. Beau's lines (following serious illness)
4. Onycholysis (thyrotoxicosis)

ABNORMAL COLOUR

1. Pallor
    (i) Anaemia
    (ii) Pale with distal brown zone (renal failure)
    (iii) Opaque white nails (hypoalbuminaemia)
2. Redness
    (i) Polycythaemia
    (ii) CO poisoning

3. Blue nails
   Cyanosis
4. Yellow nails
   Yellow nail syndrome, with lymphoedema

CAPILLARY CHANGES

1. Splinter haemorrhages
   (i) Subacute bacterial endocarditis
   (ii) Vasculitis, e.g. rheumatoid
2. Nail-fold capillary dilatation
   Collagen–vascular disease, esp. dermatomyositis, SLE

NAIL CHANGES DUE TO SKIN DISEASE

Psoriasis : pitting, onycholysis, ridging
Eczema : deformed nails with ridging
Tinea : thickened, discoloured, friable
Myxoid cyst : single groove
'Picking' at matrix : rippled grooves
Melanoma : brown or black streak (may mimic sub-lungual
            haematoma)
Erythroderma : shedding of nails

PATTERNS OF DRUG ERUPTIONS

Any drug can occasionally cause an eruption. Any eruption can
occasionally be mimicked by a drug reaction. The following list is
far from comprehensive:
1. Exanthemata (morbilliform, etc.), e.g. penicillin
2. Urticaria, e.g. penicillin
3. Erythroderma, e.g. gold
4. Bullous, including erythema multiforme, e.g. sulphonamides
5. Erythema nodosum, e.g. sulphonamides
6. Purpura (due to either thrombocytopenia or vasculitis)
7. Photosensitivity, e.g. chlorpromazine
8. Acneform (see below)
9. Fixed drug eruption (intermittent inflammation followed by
   pigmentation, always at same site), e.g. phenolphthalein

DRUGS WHICH PROVOKE AN ACNEFORM RASH

1. **B**romides and iodides
2. **A**nticonvulsants
3. **S**teroids (glucocorticoid, anabolic and androgenic)
4. **I**soniazid
5. **L**ithium
   Mnemonic: BASIL

CAUSES OF MOUTH ULCERATION

1. Aphthous ulcers
   (i) Minor
   (ii) Major
   (iii) Herpetiform
2. Squamous carcinoma (often misdiagnosed)
3. Infection, e.g. herpes simplex, syphilis
4. Lichen planus
5. Pemphigus or benign mucous membrane pemphigoid
6. Drugs, e.g. methotrexate
7. Trauma, e.g. from dentures
8. Behçet's, Reiter's or Stevens–Johnson

THREE SYSTEMIC DISEASES WHICH CAUSE CONJUNCTIVITIS WITH ULCERS OF THE MOUTH AND GENITALIA

1. REITER'S SYNDROME

Clinical features
   (i) Non-specific urethritis, haematuria, sterile pyuria
   (ii) Recurrent conjunctivitis or uveitis
   (iii) Symmetrical subacute arthritis, tenosynovitis, periostitis of ankle, knee and spine
   (iv) Circinate balanitis
   (v) Buccal ulcers
   (vi) Keratoderma blenorrhagica (resembles pustular psoriasis)

2. STEVENS–JOHNSON SYNDROME

Clinical features
   (i) Constitutional symptoms and high fever
   (ii) Conjunctivitis, corneal ulcers, uveitis
   (iii) Oral bullae and haemorrhagic crusting of lips
   (iv) Erythema multiforme
   (v) Urethritis, balanitis, vulvo-vaginitis
   (vi) Bronchitis, pneumonitis, or renal lesions

3. BEHÇET'S SYNDROME

Clinical features
   (i) Buccal and genital aphthous ulcers with a red areola
   (ii) Conjunctivitis, uveitis or retinopathy
   (iii) Cutaneous pustules, dermal nodules
   (iv) CNS lesions: meningo-encephalitis, brain-stem syndromes
   (v) Thrombophlebitis

TYPES OF PORPHYRIA

1. ACUTE INTERMITTENT PORPHYRIA

Classical triad of dark urine, abdominal pain (sometimes with nausea or constipation) and neuropsychiatric symptoms. No skin involvement

Autosomal dominant. Acute attacks provoked by drugs, e.g. oral contraceptives, alcohol, barbiturates, sulphonamides, chlorpropamide

2. PORPHYRIA CUTANEA TARDA

Photosensitivity and skin fragility. Usually develops in middle-aged patients with hepatic disease, especially alcoholic men. Associated with increased iron stores, and treated by venesection

CONDITIONS PREDISPOSING TO CANDIDIASIS

1. Skin trauma and maceration, e.g. dentures, perlèche
2. Infancy, pregnancy, old age
3. Systemic illness
   - (i) Cachexia or malignancy
   - (ii) Immunosuppression, e.g. AIDS
   - (iii) Iron deficiency
   - (iv) Endocrine disorders
     Diabetes mellitus
     Cushing's disease
     Addison's hypoadrenalism
     Hypoparathyroidism
4. Drugs
   - (i) Broad spectrum antibiotics
   - (ii) Glucocorticoids
   - (iii) Immunosuppressants

HIV AND AIDS

Group I — patients are infected with HIV and seroconvert, often with a glandular fever-like illness and rash or neurological symptoms

Group II — HIV positive patients who appear perfectly well and may remain so for many years

Group III — persistent generalized lymphadenopathy, PGL (i.e. lymphadenopathy due to reactive hyperplasia involving 2 or more sites other than the inguinal glands, and persisting for 3 or more months)

Group IV A — constitutional symptoms associated with HIV. CD4 count is greatly decreased. Clinical features include fatigue, night-sweats, lymphadenopathy, weight loss, fever, diarrhoea, etc.

Group IV B, C, D, and E are roughly equivalent to AIDS. That is the development of one or more AIDS indicator diseases for which there is no other explanation and evidence of HIV infection such as positive serology or a low CD4 count. There may be neurological disease (B), secondary infections (C), secondary cancers (D) or other conditions (E)

OPPORTUNISTIC INFECTIONS

1. Viral, e.g. cytomegalovirus, disseminated herpes simplex
2. Bacterial, e.g. atypical mycobacteria such as Mycobacteria avium–intracellulare complex
3. Fungal, e.g. systemic candidiasis, cryptococcus
4. Protozoal, e.g. Pneumocystis carinii, toxoplasmosis

MALIGNANCY IN AIDS

1. Kaposi's sarcoma
2. Lymphoma, especially cerebral

SKIN CHANGES ASSOCIATED WITH AIDS

1. Transient rash at time of seroconversion
2. Skin infections — often extensive, exaggerated, or exotic
3. Kaposi's sarcoma
4. Hairy leukoplakia of tongue
5. Many other dermatoses are commoner or more severe than in general population, e.g.:
   Seborrhoeic dermatitis
   Psoriasis
   Drug eruptions
   Xeroderma or pruritus
   Alopecia

HUMAN MALIGNANCY CAUSED BY A VIRUS (PLUS A CO-PROMOTER)

	Virus
1. Carcinoma cervix	Human papilloma virus (HPV)
2. Hepatocellular cancer	Hepatitis B
3. Nasopharyngeal cancer	EB virus (in Chinese)
4. Burkitt's lymphoma	EB virus (in malaria regions of Africa)
5. Kaposi's sarcoma	HIV plus herpes virus 8
6. T cell lymphoma	HTLV-1

13. Normal values

The International System of Units (SI units) has now been widely introduced in British laboratories in place of the traditional Imperial Units, which were empirical. Submultiples of SI units use the following prefixes:

Factor	Name	Symbol
10^{-1}	deci	d
10^{-2}	centi	c
10^{-3}	milli	m
10^{-6}	micro	μ
10^{-9}	nano	n
10^{-12}	pico	p
10^{-15}	femto	f

Even with SI units, values may vary in different laboratories

CLINICAL CHEMISTRY

Adult reference ranges — blood

Acid phosphatase: total	4–11 iu/l
prostatic	< 4 iu/l
Alanine amino-transferase (ALT)	5–45 iu/l
Albumin	35–50 g/l
Alkaline phosphatase	30–90 iu/l
Amylase	< 300 iu/l
Aspartate transaminase (AST)	10–50 iu/l
B_{12}	100–1000 ng/l
Bicarbonate	24–30 mmol/l
Bilirubin (total)	3–17 μmol/l
Corrected calcium	2.2–2.7 mmol/l*
Chloride	95–105 mmol/l
Cholesterol	3.6–6.7 mmol/l (The WHO recommends an upper limit of normal of 5.2 mmol/l for a healthier population, except in females over 60)

Cortisol: 9 am	140–690 nmol/l
12 midnight	80–190 nmol/l
C-reactive protein (CRP)	< 10 mg/l
Creatine kinase: total	< 90 iu/l
MB isoenzyme	< 6% of total
Creatinine	60–120 µmol/l
Ferritin	12–200 µg/l
Folate:	3–15 µg/l
Red cell folate	160–640 µg/l
Gamma-glutamyl transpeptidase (gamma-GT)	< 60 iu/l
Glucose (fasting)	3.6–5.8 mmol/l
Glycated haemoglobin (Hb A1c)	4.5–8%
Iron: male	14–32 µmol/l
female	10–29 µmol/l
Magnesium	0.75 –1.0 mmol/l
Osmolality	280–290 mmol/kg
Phosphate	0.8–1.4 mmol/l (i.e. approximately half of calcium)
Potassium	3.6–5.1 mmol/l
Protein (total)	60–80 g/l
Sodium	135–145 mmol/l
Thyroxine (T4): total	60–150 nmol/l
free	9–26 pmol/l
Total iron binding capacity (TIBC)	45–72 µmol/l
Triglycerides (fasting)	0.3–1.7 mmol/l
Tri-iodothyronine (T3)	1.2–3.0 nmol/l
Urea	2.5–6.6 mmol/l
Uric acid	0.1–0.4 mmol/l

HAEMATOLOGY

HAEMOGLOBIN

Men	13.0–18.0 g/dl
Women	11.5–16.5 g/dl

RED CELL COUNT (RBC)

Men	$4.5–6.5 \times 10^{12}/l$
Women	$3.9–5.6 \times 10^{12}/l$

HAEMATOCRIT (PCV)

Men	0.40–0.54
Women	0.36–0.47

* Calcium is bound to albumin and it is important to make sure that you have corrected the calcium when the albumin is abnormal. Hence:
Corrected calcium = [{40 g/l – albumin (g/l)} multiplied by 0.02] + measured calcium (mmol/l)

MEAN CELL VOLUME (MCV)

Adults 80–98 fl(cμ)

MEAN CELL HAEMOGLOBIN (MCH)

Adults 27–32 pg

MEAN CORPUSCULAR HAEMOGLOBIN CONCENTRATION (MCHC)

Adults 31–35 g/dl (g.%)

LEUKOCYTES

Adults $4–10 \times 10^9/l$
Differential: Neutrophils $2.5–7.5 \times 10^9/l$
Lymphocytes $1.5–3.5 \times 10^9/l$
Monocytes $0.2–0.8 \times 10^9/l$
Eosinophils $0.04–0.44 \times 10^9/l$
Basophils $0–0.1 \times 10^9/l$
In Black African adults, total WCC is $2.5–9 \times 10^9/l$

PLATELETS

$150–400 \times 10^9/l$

RETICULOCYTES

0.2–2%

PLASMA VISCOSITY

1.50–1.72 cp
Parallels ESR but is unaffected by age, sex or anaemia

ESR (WESTERGREN)

Men — upper limit of normal = age in years ÷ 2
Women — upper limit of normal = (age in years + 10) ÷ 2

CLOTTING TIMES

APTT   35–45 seconds
PT   10–14 seconds
INR   1

BLOOD GASES (ARTERIAL)

Oxygen 12–15 kPa (90–100 mmHg)

Carbon dioxide 4.5–6.1 kPa (34–46 mmHg)
pH 7.35–7.45
Base excess ± 2 mmol/l

URINE (ASSUMING A NORMAL DIET)

Specific gravity 1.008–1.030
pH 4.8–7.5
Protein less than 0.3 g/l
Osmolality 350–1000 mosmol/kg

CSF

Glucose, two-thirds of blood glucose value
Protein, up to 0.4 g/l
Lymphocytes, up to 4 cells/µl (i.e. 4 cells/mm^3)
Opening pressure less than 210 mm of CSF

Index